The Paleo Solution:

The Original Human Diet

ROBB WOLF

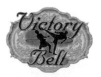

LAS VEGAS

First Published in 2010 by Victory Belt Publishing.

ISBN 10: 0-9825658-4-4

ISBN 13: 978-0-9825658-4-1

This book is for educational purposes. The publisher and author of this instructional book are not responsible in any manner whatsoever for any adverse effects arising directly or indirectly as a result of the information provided in this book. If not practiced safely and with caution, exercise can be dangerous to you and to others. It is important to consult with a professional dietitian and fitness instructor before beginning training and dieting. It is also very important to consult with a physician prior to training due to the intense and strenuous nature of the techniques in this book.

Printed in The United States

Endorsements

"I've watched as The Paleo Solution *healed people after medical professionals had given up. Whether you're an athlete, or simply uninterested in becoming a health care statistic—there are no more excuses! Now you will finally look, feel, and perform as well as your genes will allow. Robb Wolf changed my life, and he's about to change yours too."*
  —Kyle Maynard
    Author of the NY Times Bestseller *No Excuses*
    2004 ESPY Award winner

"They say the worth of a book is to be measured by what you can carry away from it. The Paleo Solution's *value is far reaching for the knowledge that it offers. Robb has taken a unique approach to health and lifestyle that will help countless people."*
  —John Welbourn
    10-Year NFL Veteran

"Robb has a rare talent for taking complex issues and conveying them to the common man. Since he is an athlete himself, he can bridge the gap between the lab coat–wearing geek scientist and competitor. On a number of occasions I've concluded one of our phone calls with "you need to write a book!" Finally it is here, the book I've wanted this terrific teacher to pen for some time now. I know that you will not only be informed, healthier, and fitter as a result of reading this work, but entertained as well."
  —Coach Michael Rutherford
    Masters National Weight Lifting Champion
    Boot Camp Fitness, Kansas City, Kansas

"Robb's guidance and advice has changed my life. Changing the way I eat has helped me stay competitive as a Crossfit athlete. There is no doubt in my mind that his food prescription was a definite factor in keeping me in the Crossfit Games "top 10" from 2007 through 2009.

"More important than athletic performance, at home the health and daily comfort of my husband, Roman, has been significantly improved upon by changing our eating habits. As an ex-boxer diagnosed with degenerative cervical disc disorder and prescribed anti-inflammatories and painkillers, he has been able to free himself of the medication through food changes.

"When I recently learned that I was pregnant, Robb was the first person I contacted for nutritional recommendations. Due to his recommendations, my body was prepared and my pregnancy has been completely free of the typical nausea and sickness. I'm thankful to have been given a small bit of Robb's vast knowledge on the topic of nutrition. That little bit has gone a long way for the health of my family."

—**Jolie Gentry**
SWAT Officer
The 2007 Crossfit Games Female Champion

"Olympic-style weightlifters, as well as many other athletes, often overlook nutrition, yet its importance cannot be taken for granted. Robb Wolf's extensive knowledge on proper nutrition and meal timing has led to an increase in performance, recovery, and overall health with numerous athletes, including myself."

—**Casey Burgener**
2008 Olympic team member, Olympic Weightlifting
2008 Gold Medal, Pan American Games

"Robb Wolf and his Paleo Solution has changed the way I look at diet and nutrition. He's helped me understand just how critical diet and sleep can be to your overall health and life."

—**Forrest Griffin**
Former UFC Light Heavyweight Champion
Author of the New York Times Bestseller *Got Fight?*

Table of Contents

Acknowledgements

I know I will forget someone, as I have so many people to thank for not only aiding in the completion of this project, but also the gym, seminars, etc. Well, here goes:

Out of the gate I need to thank Andy Deas—a great co-conspirator on the Paleolithic Solution Podcast, as well as the person who lit a fire under me to stop talking about this book and do it.

A huge acknowledgement goes to Dr. Mat Lalonde, PhD. Mat helped significantly with the technical editing of the book and made the final product so much better (scientifically accurate, readable...you name it) than it would have been. Thanks Mat.

In the science and technical theme, the following folks helped enormously by tracking down scientific journals and references: Pedro Bastos, Amy Kubal, and Brad Hirakawa.

Thanks to Yael Grauer (my "starry-eyed hippy on the street") who also helped with edits and flow.

Thanks to all of the following people who contributed work on the cover: John Welbourn, Joey Jimenez, Diane Sanfilipo, and Lou Mars. We made dozens of iterations on the cover and went some really interesting directions. John and Joey did a ton of work early on, and Diane was in the trenches tweaking the design at the 11th hour. Thanks also to the folks from Tuttle Publishing, Barnes & Noble, and Borders who offered input that I often did not want to hear, but needed to hear. I really appreciate the help all of these people gave to the project.

Thanks to Mike St. John. Brother, you are one of my best students and an inspiration. Someday I'll be "St. John Lean."

Thank you to my mentor Prof. Loren Cordain. I'm doing what I'm doing because you did what you did. I cannot thank you enough for your guidance and friendship.

Thanks to my editor, Erich Krauss, for not only taking on this project, but also for making it as important to him as it was to me. I would have never completed this project without your help.

Thanks to Glen Cordoza for your friendship and for encouraging me to take this to Victory Belt and a larger market.

To Dave Werner, Nancy Meenen, Michael Rutherford, Greg & Aimee Everett, and Chris Sommer: You have all stood by me during the toughest times in my life and have been unwavering in your friendship. This book would not be done and my life would not be what it is without you guys.

Thank you to Prof. Arthur Devany for your early guidance in my study of ancestral life-ways.

Thanks to our staff at NorCal Strength & Conditioning. I've been on the road a lot the past two years and you guys have grown and developed both the gym and yourselves.

Thank you to the many thousands of people I've met via my seminars, the blog, and podcast. This book literally is "Your" story. I would just be a chemist with a stop-watch without your support and interaction.

Thank you to Scotty Hagnas for your friendship, brainstorming, and the great meals you prepared for this book.

A garganto-thank-you to Craig "Chops" Zielinski. Without Craig's Jedi-like computer involvement I would not have a blog, the podcast, or the book. In Craig's honor, please read the entire book with a heavy Scottish accent.

And thanks finally to my wife, Nicki Violetti. I still have no idea how I roped you into marrying me, but I say a silent prayer of thanks every day we are together. Without you this book would have never taken form, and my life would lack love, fun, and adventure. You are My Girl.

Foreword

By
Prof. Loren Cordain, Colorado State University
Author of *Paleo Diet* and *Paleo Diet for Athletes*

I never thought I would laugh out loud while reading a book on Paleolithic nutrition, autoimmunity, and lipid metabolism, but I did just that while reviewing this book. With Robb being a former student of mine, it has been particularly gratifying to see the progress he has made, not only in understanding the Paleo diet for his own health needs, but also in how he turned his adversity into a passion, which has driven him to reach so many people with this life-altering message.

Who might benefit from reading *The Paleo Solution*? In a word, *everyone*. The book is peppy, upbeat, and engaging, while conveying the science and serious intent of the Paleo message. Robb has done an outstanding job of integrating vastly different disciplines in this accessible; entertaining; and, above all, practical work. It is a real tour de force, and you will love it!

You will learn about the remarkable good health of our Paleolithic ancestors, and how that health changed with the transition to agriculture and a diet dominated by humanity's "double-edged sword"—cereal grains. You will then discover how the complex interaction of our food and our hormonal system can produce either vibrant health or the many problems related to insulin dysregulation, including type 2 diabetes, cardiovascular disease, Alzheimer's, and various forms of cancer. If this wasn't enough, Robb covers not only how cereal grains underlie a host of autoimmune-related diseases, but also how they can erode your wellness by increasing inflammation in your body. You will learn a great deal about dietary fats, how the amounts and ratios of various fats have changed since our hunter-gatherer genome was established, and what this means for your health.

Possibly one of the most informative and eye-opening sections of the book deals with the stress hormone cortisol. If you are like me, you will seriously reevaluate your sleep, work, and other lifestyle variables after you read this chapter. Even if you have never exercised before, you will find the Ancestral Fitness chapter informative, instructional, and motivational. You will understand the role of exercise in maintaining your health and quality of life. Robb concludes the book with chapters addressing the practical elements of the Paleo diet: How to shop, feed the kids, a thirty-day meal plan, and a slick system for tracking your progress, which includes recommended blood work and what that blood work means.

I am fortunate to have had a significant degree of success, which has stemmed largely from my investigations in and around Paleolithic nutrition. *The Paleo Solution* is the beneficiary of this success, and via its humor and information, I suspect you will find it to be as revolutionary as it is helpful.

Prologue

I want you to try a little observation game. Go to a public location with lots of people and look around. Not in a creepy "Chester-the-Molester" way—just observe the folks around you and keep a mental tally of the following: How many people look healthy? You know, vibrant, energetic, slim, athletic. All? Some? None?

I live in Chico, California, which is famous for two things—our brewery, Sierra Nevada, and the fact that *Playboy* rated our university the "top party school in the nation" in 1987. Although our population tends to be on the younger side, we still have a decent age mix. When I play the above observation game, "How many people look healthy?" I see few examples of health. Little kids are chubby. Teenagers are muffin topped and hollow eyed. And instead of enjoying active golden years, elderly folks are consigned to walkers and wheel chairs. You may be shrugging and thinking, *Yeah, so what? That's all normal.* Well, normal can be mistaken for "common," because the above conditions are neither right nor normal.

There's an analogy about environmental change that goes like this: A frog is living in room temperature water, going about its normal froggy life. One day the temperature of the water starts to rise, but it happens so incrementally, the frog does not even notice. While he is frogging around, he literally boils alive. I'm not sure that this scenario would actually happen this way—I'd surely hope that our friend Kermit would notice things were going from balmy to bisque, but the analogy is powerful, and it eerily describes our modern world. As a society, we have become so sick, weak, and broken, we accept the *abnormal* as normal. We accept that our kids are too fat to play and blame it on "genetics." What people do not realize is that it's not a frog in the soup, it's us, and the temperature is most assuredly rising.

ONE

◇◇

My Story, Your Story, Our Story . . . (Cheezy, but true.)

◇◇

This book could save your life. No, not as a flotation device—I mean the information in it. You might have noticed from the cover that it's a "health and diet book," but it is much more than that. It is also a story as old as humanity. I know, that's a remarkably grandiose claim. At this point you have no reason to believe a word I say. I have yet to buy you a drink, and we have known each other for less than a paragraph. So, perhaps I should tell you a little bit about myself.

I grew up in Redding, California, a medium-sized town on Interstate 5, about three hours south of the Oregon border. Considering I'm a kid from rural NorCal, you might think this is a story of cow-tipping, NASCAR, and keg stands. This would reflect my heritage, and I can certainly spin a yarn about redneck shenanigans worthy of the best *Jerry Springer Show* highlight reels. But this book is not *that* story. This is the story of being the son of well-meaning, but unfortunately perpetually sick parents. Mom and Dad smoked, had heart disease, and a host of other health problems. From an early age, I was steeped in "fun" things like gall bladder surgeries, high triglycerides, pacemakers, asthma, emphysema, and arthritis. My earliest memories of my parents include a dizzying combination of medical worries, doctor visits, and medications. Not that this stuff dominated every minute of our lives, of course, but looking back now, I realize these health concerns became like background Muzak for our family.

In addition to (or perhaps because of) being sick, my parents tended to have defeatist attitudes. I remember one uplifting exchange with my mom:

Me: "What do you think it will be like when you are 100 years old?"

Mom: "Oh goodness! I hope I don't live that long!"

Me: "Why?" (A word that has defined my career path as well as landed me in hot water frequently enough to get me officially categorized as "soup stock.")

Mom's reply: "If you were that old, you would just HURT so much and you would not be able to get around. It would just be miserable."

My mom tended to be a shiny ray of sunshine. Most days.

Even at an early age, and despite the decidedly unhealthy environs of my upbringing, I had always had a notion that what we ate and how we lived could influence our health, wellness, and longevity. This innate sense, combined with my parents' poor health, spurred my interest in nutrition and fitness. I suspected that with smart food choices one need not suffer from heart disease and decrepitude. Armed with this idea, I was determined to avoid the fate of my parents.

Complementary to my interest in health and nutrition was an almost fanatical participation in the athletic activities common to most kids: football, wrestling, and karate. But as the people who know me will tell you, I tend to be obsessive about my interests. I read everything I could find on nutrition and athletic training, whether it was a book, magazine, or an old bodybuilding manual. This focus and passion for training and nutrition eventually resulted in a teenage state championship in power lifting and an amateur kick boxing record of 6-0.

I should be embarrassed to admit this, but no matter how strong my love was for athletics, it always played second fiddle to my nerdy side. In high school I competed at the state level in the Science Olympiad (Really, I did it for the girls. Really.). After high school I bounced around a number of science-related undergraduate tracks ranging from engineering to physics to molecular biology, but I eventually wrapped up a BS in biochemistry and had my sights set on medical school.

Now, this would all be fairly unremarkable were it not for the fact I also had a strong sense of rebellion and countercultural leanings. Ironically, this "dark side" led to a long deviation away from health and was nearly my undoing. You see, I developed an interest in unwashed hippy girls and vegetarianism.

Second Floor: Housewares, Vegetarianism, and Clueless Rebels

I think my story is not that different from many kids—Rebel against the basic values or norms of your parents' society. Make everything you grew up with "wrong." I thought everything American sucked, all business was evil. You know, typical youthful idiocy. It was about this time that a perfect storm of misinformation and self-delusion took my better judgment and my health from me.

The misinformation centered on the notion that vegetarianism was not only healthier than the dirty practices of eating "toxic meat," but it was morally superior as well. This certainly played to my interest in nutrition. It also sang to my youthful desire to not only be different but also live on a moral high-ground.

You may be asking yourself, "How could he let this happen?" And also "How the hell will this story save *my* life?"

I'll get to the life saving stuff in a minute. For now, you must understand my move toward vegetarianism also carried the "prize" of hippy girls. Hippy girls who tended to be both vegetarian and pretty hot. Well, "hot" in a depressed, misanthropic, high-likelihood-of-hip-fracture-due-to-a-fall sort of way. I traded in my BBQ grill for a rice steamer and pressure cooker. As a bonus, I scored a host of medical problems.

My foray into vegetarianism started innocently enough: Giant pots of steamed rice, pressure-cooked black beans, home-made hummus, and plenty of tofu-veggie stir-fry's. I'm a damn good cook, so making all this vegetarian grub taste good was *never* a problem. The problem was that my government-recommended "complex carb" meals left me ravenously hungry about forty-five minutes to an hour after eating. I also developed a monstrous sweet tooth, which I had to battle constantly. I was gassy, bloated, and started having really weird digestive problems. Looking back, I always had some problems with blood sugar swings and wacky digestion. I just assumed it was normal, especially when growing up in a house where sickness was the norm.

Interestingly, with the adoption of my vegetarian diet, these seemingly random health problems became *worse*. I studied everything I could find about vegetarian nutrition and alternative medicine. I studied at the top macrobiotic institutes, and I consulted with "experts" in vegetarian eating. After much analysis, I decided I was just detoxifying (a quasi-mythical state in which the body releases stored toxins).

So, I was vegetarian, and I "detoxed." For a few years.

When I went to the macrobiotic institute, they assured me I was on the "right track" and I just needed to "try harder." I attended yoga seminars in which vegetarian food was the topic. My problems were attributed to "moral ineptitude" and an inability to evolve! At the ripe old age of twenty-six, I had high blood pressure (140-95), high triglycerides (over 300), and bad levels of cholesterol.

The doctors at the University Health Center told me I'd need to go on blood pressure medication some day. My gambit to avoid the fate of my parents was not going well. Sick and desperate, I applied and was accepted to a school of alternative medicine. Finally, I thought, I'll get my health squared away with the knowledge I will gain at this "enlightened" institution. I'll not only be in a position to avoid the fate of my parents, but also help people find the "righteous road to health" via vegetarian living.

Academia: Abandon All Hope Ye Who Study Here

My time at the naturopathy school was a disaster. Not because of anything inherently wrong with the program, but rather because I was getting *really* sick. My high blood pressure and wacky digestion seemed inconsequential compared to a nearly crippling bout of depression that left me fixated on death every waking moment. Gross anatomy class was an intense experience with this mind-set! My stomach problems were getting worse and really scary. I went to several doctors, including naturopaths, MDs, and acupuncturists. All of them kicked things off with an abdominal exam that involved some pretty deep poking and prodding of my belly. By this stage, even mild pressure on my stomach brought about such sharp pains I would nearly leap off the table.

The MD thought I had irritable bowel syndrome and colitis. He thought I might need a bowel resection. The naturopath thought I was still detoxing. The acupuncturist was by far the most helpful and proclaimed me "a mess." I, and my health care providers, thought the diet I was eating was nearly perfect: whole grains, beans galore, tofu for protein, loads of fresh veggies. Whatever my problem, it most assuredly was not my diet! Given my dire condition: debilitating depression, colitis, high blood pressure, high triglycerides, insomnia, and a nearly constant pain throughout my body, it was the opinion of my doctors that if I were not eating as "well" as I was, I'd be dead.

I was twenty-eight years old.

I was down from a muscular and athletic 180 lbs to an emaciated 140 lbs. I literally wanted to die, but I was too big a chicken to do the deed. I was pancreas deep in the best of modern *and* alternative medicine *plus* the evolved moral thinking of the Superior Vegetarian Elite. I was screwed and I had no idea what to do. In an ironic twist, my mom's deteriorating health likely saved my life.

Go with Gut

My parents had been in and out of the hospital for surgeries, both major and minor. They had startled the family multiple times with problems so severe that we thought, *"This is it."* In the summer of 1999, my mom went in the hospital with heart and lung problems that the doctors could not get a handle on. It looked very much like these problems might kill her. The doctors said she was inflamed "everywhere." The lining of her heart and lungs seemed to be nearly on fire. She could not breathe, she was in excruciating pain. It's nothing you want to see anyone go through, especially your mom.

The only thing that seemed to help was high doses of anti-inflammatory drugs, but these had powerful side effects nearly as bad as her original problem. This went on for days, until finally a diagnosis was made: Autoimmune disease. My mom's immune system, designed to protect her from microbial invaders like bacteria and viruses, had turned on her and appeared hell-bent on killing her. When the medical reports came back, we were stunned, as she had a laundry list of interconnected diseases: rheumatoid arthritis, systemic lupus erythematosus, Sjögren's syndrome. I'd heard of some of these, others were completely new to me.

With the diagnosis came a treatment plan involving immune-suppressing drugs and anti-inflammatories. These drugs were dangerous and prone to complications, but the cocktail would at least quiet the warfare in her body to a point that she would live and be reasonably comfortable. Amid this fear, confusion, and drama, a quiet discovery was made by some routine lab work ordered by the rheumatologist: In addition to the autoimmune diseases, my mom also had an intolerance to a protein called gluten, which is found in wheat, oats, rye, barley, and a few other grains. The disease is called celiac, and, as I mentioned, this diagnosis likely saved my life.

A phone call with my mom revealed that her celiac disease was a type of autoimmune response in the small intestine. She told me many people suffered from the problem with varying degrees of severity. Her rheumatologist suspected that the celiac might be at play in all of her autoimmune conditions. The solution was simple in theory, nearly impossible in practice: remove all foods that contain gluten from the diet: bread, pasta, most cereal, and all sorts of baked goods. Sauces, marinades, and similar prepared items are suspect too, as everything seems to contain gluten in one form or another. Not only do you need to read labels, you have to be exceptionally careful while eating out. A grilled chicken breast could be contaminated with gluten by simply being cooked on a grill that had shared French bread from an earlier meal.

For my mom, the removal of gluten brought an immediate improvement in her stomach issues and autoimmune condition. She had suffered from gall stones years before, and this lead eventually to the removal of her gall bladder. She had also suffered from the same problems as I had: colitis, acid reflux, and the catch-all term "irritable bowel syndrome" (IBS). Interestingly, my mom's rheumatologist also recommended she avoid most legumes, such as beans and bean sprouts, as they were known to irritate conditions such as lupus and rheumatoid arthritis.

This was happy news for me because my mom was feeling better (although still far from healthy), but it was also a world-altering moment. My mom's illness and presumably *my* illness was *caused* by the holiest of holies: the vegetarian diet. The base of the food pyramid! Grains and legumes, the most wholesome and righteous of foods, appeared to be out to kill us.

I was stunned. How could this be? If whole grains and legumes were making us sick, what should I eat? I was literally sitting on my doorstep on an uncharacteristically warm and sunny day in Seattle when an idea struck me: How did we evolve? What did we eat in our remote past? Hunter-gatherers, evolutionary biology: the Paleo diet. I remembered hearing about a way of eating that emulated the diets of our hunter-gatherer forebears.

I jumped up and went in the house, turned on the computer (waited forever for the dial-up to engage), and used a nifty new search engine called Google to research the term "Paleo diet." What I found stunned me. Our human and prehuman ancestors had lived for 3 million years with a remarkably high level of health, eating only lean meats, seafood, nuts, seeds, and seasonal fruits and vegetables. The agricultural "revolution" saw our ancestors become small, weak, and sick. Infant mortality exploded.

The most important site I found initially was Professor Arthur Devany's *Evolutionary Fitness*. Professor Devany is a retired economist who has emulated the exercise and eating of a hunter-gatherer for over thirty years. He is seventy years old, six feet two inches tall, and 205 lbs with less than 10 percent body fat. This was the normal state for our hunter gatherer forebears. I began corresponding with Prof. Devany and, at his suggestion, I contacted Prof. Loren Cordain of Colorado State University, who would ultimately become my mentor in the study of Paleolithic nutrition.

Professor Cordain was the world's leading expert on the topic of ancestral diet as it relates to our health and wellness. His research was published in journals ranging from immunology to rheumatology to ophthalmology to nutrition. This is unheard of in the modern world of scientific specialization. His secret? If you know the answer (evolutionary biology) it is easy to reverse engineer the question. Prof. Cordain knew that evolution via natural selection was the answer to modern health questions.

Other key resources in my early learning included the books *Protein Power* and *Protein Power: LifePlan* by Michael and Mary Eades. The Eades had worked as bariatric physicians for over twenty years. Their amazing success with overweight patients was the result of understanding our ancestral diet. They reversed diabetes, depression, GI problems, and autoimmunity while helping clients lose enormous amounts of weight.

What's Old Is New

What I learned flew in the face of everything I'd studied about vegetarianism. Protein and fat were not bad; carbohydrates meant fruits and veggies, not bagels and rice. I had two competing worldviews as diametrically opposed as the Cold War struggle of communism and capitalism, and I had only one thing left to do:

Try it.

But I had huge reservations. I was confident I'd followed the vegetarian prescription precisely. I knew how to cook and mix meals, and I had been diligent in my efforts to eat a perfect vegetarian diet. However, my only rewards thus far were rapidly declining health and frustration. As a result, I pushed my reservations aside and went shopping.

I bought a pack of ribs from Whole Foods, along with salad fixings. I made a rub of garlic and ginger powder for the ribs and set them baking in the oven. I made a salad of field greens, fennel, and sweet red onions. Two hours later, the timer on the oven rang, and I reset it for twenty minutes to let the meat "rest" (which seemed odd considering it was already dead). When the second timer rang, I cut off a section of ribs and piled my plate high with salad. I garnished the whole mess with olive oil and balsamic vinegar. I ate. And ate, and ate. About six ribs and a pound of salad later I was warmly satisfied, clear headed, and I felt better than I had in years.

After one meal.

I had no gas, no bloat, and no stomach problems. That night I slept better than I had in recent memory. I woke up the next day rested and not in a fog. I made scrambled eggs with chopped basil and rounded things out with half a cantaloupe. I felt great! I had energy, I could think. I actually felt like I wanted to *live*.

I ran with this for two weeks, feeling better and better. I immediately lost the layer of chub that had grown around my midsection despite the fact that I was emaciated. I started gaining muscle and losing fat at the same time. I went to the doctor for a scheduled checkup on my colitis and reported that I felt great, symptom free! The doctor performed his standard abdominal exam and remarked that I was not levitating off the table due to pain. I told him I had completely changed my diet, switching to lean meats, fruits, and veggies.

"Doc! Have you ever heard of the Paleo diet?" I asked. "How our ancestors ate for millennia?"

His answer was typical of what I would encounter in the years to follow. "That is pseudo science. There is no proof."

I went home and ate "pseudo science" for breakfast, lunch, and dinner. I felt better than I ever had in my life. I gave away my rice cooker and felt bad because I knew I should just smash the thing. I went in for another checkup, this time with my general practitioner to check my blood work. I was in for a shock right from the beginning: blood pressure—115/60. My normal for years had been 140/90. At this point, I'd been eating Paleo for about six weeks. When my blood work came back, my doctor and I were beside ourselves. Triglycerides were down from over 300 to 50. My formerly low "good" HDL cholesterol was up, my "bad" LDL cholesterol was way down. The doctor asked what I'd changed.

"I started eating a Paleo diet. I feel great!" I said. "Everything has changed!"

The doctor's only remark was, "It must be something else."

Thanks Doc!

The change in my health and the lack of interest on the parts of my health care providers prompted me to pull the plug on studying medicine, alternative or otherwise. I went into research and studied how different fats affect diseases such as cancer and diabetes. Remarkably, everyone in the lab was on a Paleo diet when I arrived! These folks had tracked their blood work for years and knew that too much refined carbs would start moving blood markers of disease in the wrong direction.

I enjoyed this work, but I missed seeing people and working around health and fitness (lab work is not the place for the extroverted, energetic person I discovered). I concocted the wild idea of moving back to my old Northern California college town, Chico, to open a gym of all things and start helping people to live longer, better lives.

Ten Years? It Didn't Feel a Day over Twenty!

Fast forward ten years. I'm co-owner of NorCal Strength & Conditioning, a highly successful gym that was picked by the editors of *Men's Health* as one of the "top thirty gyms in America." I have a popular and high-traffic blog that explores how a Paleo diet plus smart exercise can improve performance, health, and longevity. I cofounded the magazine the *Performance Menu* as a means of reaching more people with the message of Paleolithic nutrition. I also travel the world providing lectures in optimizing performance and health. I have about 30,000 e-mails from people living all around the world that I've worked with in some capacity testifying to the fact that Paleo nutrition has transformed their lives. People with cancer, diabetes, heart disease, and autoimmunity have all benefited from Paleo nutrition. We have produced world-champion athletes in sports as disparate as mixed martial arts (MMA) to triathlon and motocross. We have helped hundreds of people in our gym by educating them on sound nutrition and providing the framework for fun, challenging workouts.

I do not relate this to you to be boastful. Quite the contrary, this has little or nothing to do with me other than I asked these many thousands of people to do the scariest thing imaginable: Take a chance, give a Paleo diet a shot. Dare to turn back the hands of time and live the full genetic potential with which we are born into this world. What started off as "my" story of health and wellness has become the story of thousands. I'd like to share a few of these interesting and inspiring stories with you.

Testimonials

Glen Cordoza, mixed martial artist

My search for the perfect diet began about seven years ago. I was preparing for my first professional mixed martial arts fight and was trying to clean up my diet in hopes that it would increase my performance. At this time, my knowledge of nutrition was rudimentary at best. I had taken a nutrition class in college and my instructor had stressed whole grains, pastas, and rolled oats as my primary food sources. In short, the food guide pyramid served as my platform for healthy eating.

Although this seemed to work, I knew that there was more out there and sought other diets. I tried virtually everything under the sun. While spending a year in Thailand competing as a professional Muay Thai kickboxer, my diet shifted from breads and pastas to rice, and I seemed to get good results. I thought that my nutrition was pretty much dialed. That was of course before I met nutrition guru Robb Wolf.

Robb and his approach to the Paleo diet have changed my life. Like most people that have been sold on the food guide pyramid or other diets that stress whole grain products, I met the Paleo diet with harsh criticism. I questioned everything, and was highly skeptical. I mean, who was this guy telling me that whole wheat and grains are bad for you? It went against everything that I've been taught. He told me the benefits that I would receive and suggested that I try it out for a month to see if worked. I did, and almost immediately I felt like a new man.

No longer doubting his teachings, Robb helped break down every aspect of my diet, including portion size based on my body composition and work output, pre- and postworkout nutrition, intermittent fasting, and insulin sensitivity. Now that I have been a student of his for two years, I no longer consider Paleo a diet. It has become a lifestyle.

The advantages linked to the Paleo diet cannot be overstated. My life in and out of the gym has changed dramatically. I've seen a continuous increase in all areas of my performance; I'm leaner, stronger, faster, and my recovery is phenomenal. Outside of the gym, I have seen a dramatic increase in my productivity level. I've coauthored over ten books and I'm getting twice as much work done in half the amount of time. I know this might sound absurd, but it's the honest truth. My sleep has improved, food tastes better, my stress levels have dropped (oh man, have they dropped), I have more energy throughout the day, I seldom get sick, and my allergies have completely subsided. Thanks to the teachings of Robb Wolf, I feel better than I ever thought imaginable. With such miraculous benefits, I am absolutely certain that this is the optimum diet.

Author's Note:

Glen came to us as a high-level athlete, fresh off a sixteen month stint doing professional Thai boxing bouts in Thailand. He was a fit, muscular, 162 pounds, and he had thirteen percent body fat. When we put him to the test with strength and conditioning, he had impressive performance to say the least. By all appearances, his rice-based, Thai diet was working wonders for him. However, with a little arm-bending (which with Glen is a really difficult thing to accomplish), we convinced him to give Paleo a shot. Nine months later, Glen was a shredded 175 pounds with seven to eight percent body fat. He could clean and jerk 275 pounds (this is lifting the weight from floor to overhead in two quick movements), and had crushing work-capacity when fighting. Glen usually fights at 155 pounds, and although our modifications would seem like it moved him in the wrong direction, the Paleo diet actually made it easier for him to cut weight leading up to, and the night before, competition. It also made it easier for him to put that weight back on the morning of the fight. What this translates into is eighteen pounds of additional muscle when he stepped into the ring. Due to the Paleo diet, he was larger and stronger than the opponents he went up against, despite still falling into the 155 pound weight class. Now, almost four years later, Glen is both physically and vocally one of our strongest advocates of the Paleo Solution.

Dr. James Curtis, DDS

I was sixty-nine years old and had been following popular diets for about fifteen years with a serious lack of success. I had yo-yoed from 235 pounds to 201 pounds and back to 225 pounds, which I maintained for about ten years. My blood pressure was high and stayed around 140/89. Eventually this deteriorated physical state led to two heart stents about two years ago. My medication list was impressive:

Lotensin 80mg
Atenolol 50mg
Plavix 75mg
Norvasc 10mg
Lipitor 40mg

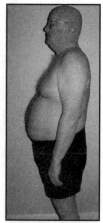

February 1, 2007

I attended the Robb Wolf Paleo Seminar on January 31, 2007, and have done the Paleo diet religiously ever since. After six months of his program, my blood panel is *perfect*. I am off of all medications except for Lotensin 40mg, and Norvasc 5 mg. I think my doctor won't take me off the rest of the meds for fear I won't come back to see him!

My blood pressure is now 115/69, while my weight is now 176 pounds and dropping slowly. I am looking at another 10 to 15 pounds before I reach a healthy maintenance weight.

I have been doing CrossFit since April 15 of 2008, but am only up to the puppies workouts. You can't fool mother nature. Sixty-nine years old is still sixty-nine years old. I am Level I certified and have a garage gym. I quote Robb directly, "Exercise is important, but diet is critical."

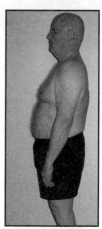

My carbs are mostly salad and stir-fry veggies. Lots of eggs, chicken, beef, and shrimp. I have my own chickens and cows. I have a little fruit for a snack. I am never hungry and sometimes have to make myself eat. Because of Robb's plan, I now have a life instead of waiting to die. How do you thank someone for that?

May 1, 2007

Authors Note:

Dr. Curtis attended my nutrition seminar and attacked the program with a vengeance. He maintains a full dental practice but made no excuses. He preps his meals ahead of time or makes smart choices while eating out. He acted with dedication and look at the results. I suspect the Paleo Solution can extend one's life, but I have no proof of that. Yet. What I can prove is that it adds life to the years we have. Regardless of age or current health status, we can affect remarkable change in our quality of life—you just need to want a better life more than the perceived comforts of poor nutrition and an unhealthy lifestyle. That choice is yours. No matter how good the program, it still comes down to you.

Sarah Fragoso, strength coach, mother of three

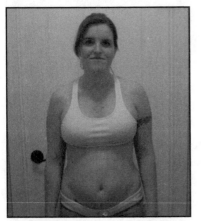

February 1, 2008

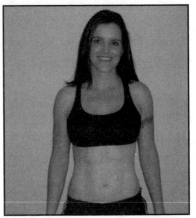

September 1, 2008

After my third son was born (yes, I have three boys . . .) I was overjoyed, but also fat and exhausted. I always had a lot of energy, even during my pregnancy, but I had begun to notice toward the end of my pregnancy that I was tired above and beyond the norm. Furthermore, the swelling in my legs, although not visibly horrible, was extremely painful to the touch, and even weeks after my son was born, the swelling did not go away. My husband tried to rub my legs, but I could hardly stand his touch. I felt trapped in my lethargic, overweight, unhappy body, and as wonderful as it was to have my new little one, I had zero energy for my other two.

A month rolled by and nothing was better. I found myself in tears at the end of each day, feeling like a failure and hating that the only thing I could fit into was my husband's sweat pants. Two months after the baby, I had lost a little of the weight but my energy was still zapped. I thought I had a handle on my nutrition, eating lots of whole grains, vegetables, and good protein, but I stepped back and looked at my food intake and noticed that there was more sugar, processed foods, and pasta on my plate than what I had imagined I was eating.

I knew I needed to make a change, and although I wasn't sure at that point that the big change I needed to make was my food, the fact that I could not keep up with my life had me convinced that something needed to be done. I was done being tired, grumpy, swollen, and sore. Done being fat, burnt out, and stressed. Done wondering what I should do and ready to find a real solution.

So, three months after giving birth to my third son, and after many nights of crying and frustration, I made a change. One freezing February morning at six o'clock, my husband took out his sweat pants for me, handed me my giant sports bra, made me pump a bottle of breast milk, and kicked me out of the house for my first workout with Robb Wolf at NorCal Strength & Conditioning. I never looked back. Yes, working out was amazing and I could write another whole story about that, but what I learned about food from Robb is really what changed, or should I say, saved my life.

After a few weeks of the crazy six AM workouts, I asked Robb how I could look better and feel better faster, and he introduced me to the Paleo way of eating. I promised I would give it a go for thirty days, willing at this point to try anything, and in two short weeks, despite my nights moaning on the couch for ice cream and French bread, the first thing I noticed was that the terribly painful swelling in my legs was totally gone. Not just better, but gone!

This alone was enough to convince me that Paleo eating was worth giving up the grains and sugar, worth thinking ahead, and worth the extra degree of effort to make sure I had enough food on hand to avoid driving my carload of crazed kids into the nearest drive thru.

After three months, I tossed the hubby's sweats, squeezed into some old workout pants I hadn't worn in years, and went to my next six AM workout. Robb's awesome wife, Nicki, told me I looked sexy—and I was even more convinced!

Seven short months later I was a different person. I wasn't back to my pre-baby body, I was *better* than that. More fit, lean, muscular, clear-headed, and healthier than I had ever been in my life. Furthermore, I had figured it out. Eating Paleo, eating clean, eating how our bodies are intended to eat, is not hard—it just makes sense. I simply had to retrain my body to eat the kinds of foods we are supposed to eat rather than what we are sold by the media as "good" nutrition.

After a year of Paleo eating, I had rid my house entirely of non-Paleo food items and my three kids and husband had jumped on the Paleo band wagon (In reality, I tied them all up and threw them on the wagon, but they survived and are better for it!). I now really notice when my kids eat non-Paleo food items. Time spent at friends' houses or with Grandpa leaves them grumpy, sugar-dosed little monsters.

My oldest, who is now fourteen, was the hardest to convince when it came to eating Paleo, but now he is old enough to notice the difference in how he feels when he eats processed foods. Luckily, he loves cooking and is always in the kitchen, preparing new Paleo meals. He has even started writing down his own recipes in hopes of opening his own Paleo restaurant someday.

Overall, I am so grateful that I found a way to not only be healthy, but to also be well. I know that I am doing all I can to protect myself and my family from modern-day diseases, and I know that I am giving my family the best gift I can—a mother who really loves being a mother, has energy at the end of the day, and knows she can wake up in the morning to do it all over again (and worth noting, my husband is oh so glad that I no longer fit into his sweat pants).

Authors Note:

In Sarah's initial seven-month period of training with us, she lost over thirty-five pounds of scale weight and went from a size fourteen to a size two. After a year, she was down to a size zero. As impressive as that is, it's important to keep in mind that she gained some muscle and thus her fat loss was likely in the 40–45 pounds range. She progressed from having no pull-ups to fifteen to twenty pull-ups. She also progressed from being unable to lift a 65-pound barbell off the floor to lifting a 220-pound barbell that was nearly double her body weight. This is a lesson to you women who are afraid to lift weights for fear of "getting too big." If you want to look, feel, and perform your best, you need to get strong and eat well. This has worked for the 10,000 women that I have trained, so you can keep doing it your way or try "our" way.

Their Story Becomes Your Story

I don't want this to become an infomercial. The ShamWOW guy can put me into a kind of catatonic drooling state similar to my college drinking days, and I do not want to do that to you. I *do* want to impress upon you that everyone will benefit from a Paleo diet, plus smart exercise and lifestyle tweaks: Olympic-caliber athletes, stay-at-home moms, grandparents, and folks who, unfortunately, might be very sick.

Oftentimes, we hear the question, "Will this approach work for me?" to which I offer the Zen-flavored answer: "Only if you *do* it." I wish I could make a program that allowed people to eat crap foods, never exercise, skip sleep, and still be healthy and look good. It won't happen. Not out of a box or from a pill. You *will* need to change a few things.

The media, talk shows, and unscrupulous venders of fads dress up the same inaccurate messages that guarantee frustration and failure. It's a great racket: Sell you something that does not work and blame you for the failure! What I have to offer cuts the cycle of fads, pills, and potions that do not work and puts you 100 percent in charge of your destiny and results. It is your call as to what level of buy-in you give this. For some, the prospect of looking and feeling great is enough to affect change. For others, it's not. It's your call what camp you want to be in. What I'm presenting here, however, is money in the bank: *If you make a few minor changes to your eating and lifestyle, you will see a stunning return on investment.* Better results than anything else you have ever tried. Bold statement? Yes it is, and all you need to do to either succeed or prove me wrong is give it a shot.

Knowledge Is Power

Now, I come from a scientific background, so I tend to like the geeky stuff. This book will provide you the opportunity to learn a lot. You may be surprised, but learning a little will not ruin your social life or doom you to wearing a pocket protector. You will learn why so many people in our modern society of plenty are sick with diseases we rarely if ever saw in the past: cancer, depression, Parkinson's, Alzheimer's, diabetes, heart disease, and autoimmunity. You will learn why eating a diet and living a lifestyle at odds with our genetic heritage is shortening lives and costing us millions, even billions, of dollars as a society. You will learn how to change your nutrition and lifestyle to not only restore health and vigor, but to also reverse the ravages of time. Old age need not be a time of decrepitude and misery. You will learn how to make incremental changes that are simple and easy to live with.

Thousands of people have made this change and love the results, and so will you. For those of you less concerned with health and longevity than with "looking good *neked*," don't despair, you will get your goods as well. The reality is our genetic heritage *wants* us to look good.

In contrast to the modern prescriptions for weight loss that involve starvation, pills, and potions that damage our health and fail to work, we will tap into our hunter-gatherer genetics to look, feel, and perform our best. I will draw upon anthropology, genetics, and biochemistry to explain a little bit of the "whys." After all, many people need a little convincing before they jump into a new program. God love the type of folks who think! For others, they just want to know how to do it and how to know if they are doing it right. I've got all that covered.

Whoever you are, whatever your situation, what I need from you is simple: Give it a shot for thirty days. I will provide simple, effective methods of tracking progress—you just need to do it! For some of you this will be an easy transition, for others, I can't lie, it's going to be tough, but you will all benefit from these simple changes and in ways you cannot imagine.

Just to give you a sense of where we are going, in the next chapter we will look at our hunter-gatherer past so we can understand our natural birthright of health and vitality. Then we will begin to learn why everyone is so sick and discover how "high insulin levels from the wrong carbohydrates," "a breakdown in the digestive process," and "an imbalance of essential fats" are conspiring to undermine our health and longevity. We will also look at lifestyle and stress and their roles in looking and feeling our best. We will then shift into the "How To" section, which will show you how to hunt and gather your nutrition from the modern mega-food chaos. We will look at how to prep food, eat on the go, and make the best of bad food situations. Then we will look at exercise and lifestyle from a Stone Age perspective. You might be a little jealous of how our Paleolithic ancestors lived! We will also look at feeding and watering the family unit. Folks love to make the topic of kids far more complicated than it needs to be—I'll help you keep it simple and effective for the kiddos.

If you are the short-attention-span type, you can jump right to the prescriptive chapters. You do not need to know "why" to be able to "do." You can always read up on a specific chapter later, as you are likely to get a lot of questions about how you started looking and feeling so much better. Just remember, though, if you have questions, the answers *are* in the book. For the contrarians out there, I have a thorough reference section, and I address common counterpoints both in the appendix and throughout the book. But instead of wasting my time and yours, just get in and give this a shot. My motivation is simple: I'm trying to save your life. I never could help my parents—it would sure be nice if you'd let me help *you*.

TWO

<><><><><><><><><><><><><><><><><><><><><><><><><><><><><><>

Hunter Gatherers Are Us
Or
You Can Take the Kid Out of the Savannah, but You Can't Take the Savannah Out of the Kid!

<><><><><><><><><><><><><><><><><><><><><><><><><><><><><><>

This book is a story about us. You know, *H. Sapiens*. It's also a story of how to optimize our performance, health, and longevity. While combining such monumental plot lines might lead you to believe this is one of those family saga novels that jumps all over in time, don't worry. This story both starts and ends in the past. However, in order to fully appreciate this story, it is important to replace your current view of "time" with that of certain ancient cultures. The ancients' view of time worked something like this:

You are in the middle of a river (Time) and facing downstream. The future approaches you from behind . . . only to recede into the past, which actually lies in front of you, moving ever farther away. If you could look far enough downstream you would see the beginning of the stream and, in essence, everything.

This may seem odd and difficult to imagine at first, but as you get deeper into this book, not only will this philosophy make more sense, but you will also see that it is a more accurate description of reality.

Think about it like this: Our current worldview is like the "crazy guy" at the bus station. He gets through life, but not very effectively. Once you have a more realistic, past-centric orientation, you will be able to make sense of modern health and disease. And perhaps quit scaring people at the bus stop.

Stop! Savannah Time!

It is our natural birthright to be fit and healthy. Unfortunately, science and medicine have largely missed this point. Researchers look boldly to the future, to new medicines, genetic screening, and surgical procedures, yet never ask the questions, "Why do we need these advances?" and "Is there a simpler, better way to health and wellness?" If they were to ask these questions, they would realize that the key to the puzzle is to start at the beginning. Our health researchers, who currently lack a framework from which to assess the staggering volume of information they generate every day, flounder with basic questions: "What should we eat?" "How much and what types of exercise should we do?" "How can we live a healthy life?" Although these may seem like sound questions for health researchers to ask, the answers constantly change in response to politics, lobbying, and the media. As a result, their recommendations are *not* based on science, but rather lobbying and political maneuvering.

Our system is confused and broken, and we are being held hostage by an Orwellian nutrition and health research community that lacks a unifying theory to assess the validity of one study over another. They do not even know where to start looking for answers, which makes our "health maintenance system" more parasitic than symbiotic. The worst part is that few people make a real attempt to fix this mess. But who can really blame them. After all, it's hard as hell to make money off healthy people . . . unless you sell bicycles, running shoes, or teach dance classes.

Is this debacle making any sense? Let me provide an analogy to help explain it a little better. Imagine you have a box full of ceramic fragments, half of which are green and half of which are red. It is your task to put these pieces back together to form the complete, original object. Now, let's imagine two scenarios. In the first scenario, you know the object you must construct is a bowl composed of only the red ceramic shards. In the second scenario, you have no idea what the object is, and besides that, you must wear glasses that make all the pieces, both red and green, look brown. Do you think it might be tough to complete this task if every bit of information (the ceramic pieces) looked essentially the same and you had no real idea of what you were trying to construct? I think it's obvious this would be a damn confusing and frustrating situation. Well, it happens to be analogous to our state of affairs in the nutritional sciences, medicine, and most of health research. Everyone has blinders on, every study looks as good as any other, and we have no unifying theory from which to assess our findings. As a result, you constantly receive different information on what is healthy and what is not. One year eggs will save your life, and the next they will put you into the grave.

Need a more concrete example of how this is affecting you? Here is a good one:

Fat Makes You Fat, Right?

Oddly enough, no. Epidemiologists are befuddled by why fat does not make us fat. Ever hear of the French Paradox? Spanish Paradox? The French (and Spanish, and Sardinians, and Greeks) eat far more fat than Americans (while consuming a fraction of the *sugar*) yet do not get fat, diabetic, or cancerous at the rates we do. Why? Our dieticians tell us we eat too many calories and too much fat. Fat has nine calories per gram, while carbohydrate and protein only have four! Obviously the "fat makes us fat" paradigm is right, isn't it? Don't we just need to eat less and make "sensible" food choices? Isn't this all just a matter of willpower? Does my inner child need a spanking because I fell off *another* high-carb, low-fat diet? Most people try these "sensible" approaches, fail, and end up fatter, sicker and more despondent than before. Why do all the buzz words of dietitians (willpower, moderation, manifesting, balance, fiber, counting calories) fail?

Why?

What explains this? Unfortunately, the answer to this question requires yet another question: Are there examples of people who *do not* suffer from the scourges of cancer, autoimmunity, obesity, diabetes and neurodegeneration? The answer ironically is "yes," there are people who live free of these diseases. However, when presented with this information, most doctors, dieticians, and researchers ignore it because it challenges the paradigm in which they garb themselves. Little do they know it's a case of the Emperor's New Clothes. Our medical community is naked. So, it's back to more studies comparing a 15 percent fat diet with a 20 percent fat diet, all with 55–60 percent carbs from whole grains, because everybody knows you would fall over and die without your bran muffin.

Perhaps I should not be so hard on our research community. After all, those pointless studies are good for keeping departments of universities open and well funded. But oddly enough, I am more interested in saving you than keeping these goofballs funded and in tenure-track positions. In order to accomplish this goal of saving your fanny, I must help you face the music, and the song is an old one.

Don't Confuse Me with the Truth

One might think that people (nutrition scientists included) would find solace in understanding how powerfully our genetic heritage influences both our present *and* future. But quite to the contrary, this idea generates a remarkable amount of resistance. The answer is *too* simple, and it annoys some folks that the answers to most of life's ills lie in our past. For others, it's uncomfortable to realize that we, *H. Sapiens*, are a part of nature.

We, like all critters great and small, are bound by our heritage on this planet. This fact has a way of undermining our sense of "beautiful flower" uniqueness, but really it should not. We just need to shift our focus from upstream to downstream and appreciate our remarkable heritage. We (you and me) represent an unbroken lineage of life that extends back to the dawn of time. Pretty cool, no?

Some of you are on board with all this, some are not. Good; don't believe a thing I say. Instead try what I recommend in the "how-to" section of the book and see if you look, feel, and perform better. That's a fair proposition, right? Once you see that the Paleo Solution works, you will likely want to know "why." To address the "whys," I will build my case throughout the book starting from mechanistic descriptions of disease. You will learn exactly how our modern life causes diabetes, autoimmunity, cancer, neurodegeneration, and infertility. Then you will learn how to avoid or reverse these ills.

Before we get to all that science, I want to look at a little anthropology. Considering I was a biochemist by trade before becoming a strength coach, you might think I would be swayed more by the mechanisms and pathology presented later. I'm not. It's important for me to cover that material, as it helps you and your doctor make sense of how a Paleo approach can improve your health and reverse disease, but, even as a geek, I find the mechanisms and pathology tedious and a little boring. In stark contrast, the anthropology and historical aspects of this story touch something in me besides the intellect, and it *moves* me. Instead of metabolic pathways, genetics, and biochemistry, we consider living, breathing people and how their diet affected their way of life. This is a microcosm of the world-changing shift all of our ancestors made. A change from millions of years of the hunter-gatherer way of life to the ultimate global experiment: agriculture.

As you will see, this change has been a Faustian bargain, and the Devil has not finished taking his due. Not convinced? Let's have a few drinks in my hometown of Chico, California, and talk with the experts on this topic.

Agriculture: Get In Early! It's the Next Big Thing! Unlimited Growth Potential! Work from Home!

Chico, California, is a great little college town. The campus is beautiful and partially encircled by the quaint downtown business area. There are a number of great eateries and bars, just the place to do an undergraduate degree in four to seven years. Now, let's imagine you came to Chico and we went out for a lunch of shrimp cocktails and NorCal margaritas. Its 11 AM. We have been talking Paleo nutrition throughout the lunch (I know, big yawn, hang with me here) and you are 100 percent tipsy but only 50 percent convinced on this "Paleo diet" thing. You admit that I can spin a damn convincing yarn, but you want to bounce some ideas off folks who are not "zealots" like me. I suggest that we go to the experts on this topic, as the Department of Anthropology is only a short walk across campus.

"Anthropology?" you ask. "Shouldn't we go to the Nutritional Sciences Department?"

I smile. "Sure, but we will hit that *after* the Anthropology stop."

We finish our margaritas (waste not, want not) and embark on our adventure. As luck would have it, most of the Anthropology Department is eating lunch together this day. When we walk in, someone asks, "Can we help you?"

"We need Anthropologists," I respond. "Now!"

We do not look too dangerous, so these folks invite us to have a seat and to explain what we need. I want to do this in a way that is not leading, as you are only half convinced of this Paleo-craziness, and I ponder my first question carefully. Finally I ask, "What is the single most important event in all of human history? What changed things, for good or ill, more than any other event or occurrence?"

A low murmur builds amid the faculty as they begin weighing potential answers. This goes on for a minute or so before the room quiets and the department chair, a stately woman in her early fifties, announces, "The agricultural revolution." All heads around the table nod agreement. Your head nods because of the margaritas, but you are drawn in by the consensus. You are not completely out of it, however, and ask an important follow-up question.

"Why? Why is the agricultural revolution so important?"

The faculty murmurs briefly and, again, the department chair replies. "Let's look at this question in a way that paints human history in a relative scale. If we stood on an American football field (100 yards from end-zone to end-zone) we could represent a timeline of human history in the following way: If we started walking from one end-zone toward the other, we could walk 99.5 yards, and this would represent all of human history except the last 5,000 years or so. . . 99.5 of the 100 yards.

"This is when our genetics were selected for survival in a hunting-gathering lifeway and we were damn good at it. We evolved and adapted to this way of living and the interaction of our genetics and our environment made us who we were, and who we *are*. Our genetics are virtually identical to those of our early human ancestors from more than 120,000 years ago. The last 10,000 years, the time in which we transitioned from the hunting and gathering lifeway to agriculture, is the last half yard of our timeline. The last few inches represent television, the Internet, refined vegetable oils, and most of what we take to be "normal" modern living."

The room falls silent and it's obvious the department head and the rest of the group are waiting for a response. You are taking all this in and ask another important question. "What happened with this change healthwise? What were we like as hunter-gatherers, and what happened when we changed to agriculture?"

A new surge of discussion, and then the department chair starts in again. "Oh, that's a great question! Our HG ancestors were remarkably healthy. They were as tall or taller than modern Americans and Europeans, which is a sign they ate a very nutritious diet. They were virtually free of cavities and bone malformations that are common with malnutrition. Despite a lack of medical care, they had remarkably low infant mortality rates, yet had better than 10 percent of their population live into their sixties.

"Historical accounts of contemporary HGs who were studied by explorers and anthropologists show these people to be virtually free of degenerative disease such as cancer, diabetes, and cardiovascular disease. They also showed virtually no near-sightedness or acne. Our HG ancestors were powerfully built, with strength and endurance on a par with modern athletes. This fitness was built by living the foraging lifestyle, which was active yet afforded much downtime and relaxation. Most people contributed about ten to fifteen hours per week toward food, clothing, and shelter, with the remaining time spent talking, visiting family members in nearby groups, or simply resting."

You take this in. It's interesting, almost convincing, but you have watched your share of Discovery Channel and you seem to recall HGs lived short brutish lives. You articulate as much to the group and you add that it's seems like a remarkable assortment of "just-so" stories, all this talk of "tall cave men with good teeth." You ask a pointed question: "Isn't this all a bunch of conjecture? Why don't I hear about this more if it's true?"

The department chair looks at her colleagues, shrugs, and then motions toward the floor to ceiling books and journals lining the walls. "These are all accounts of early peoples. Hunter-gatherers, pastoralists, and agriculturalists have been extensively studied since the mid-1800s.

We know quite a lot about how these people lived, what they ate, and the relative differences in their health and wellness. The whole field of forensic science is an outgrowth of medical anthropology. Are you aware that a trained forensic scientist or medical anthropologist can tell you within minutes whether an ancient skeleton was that of a hunter-gatherer or agriculturalist? This based on the remarkably increased rates of dental caries (cavities), bone malformations, and general poor health of the early farmers as compared to their hunter-gatherer cousins."

You are becoming more convinced by the second, but you want something more tangible. "Do you have any specific examples of this difference you could show me?"

The department chair thinks a moment, then excuses herself and heads to her office. In a few minutes she returns with an old, well-worn book titled, *Nutritional Anthropology: Contemporary Approaches to Diet and Culture*. She turns to a chapter called "Nutrition and Health in Agriculturalists and Huntergatherers: A Case Study of Two Pre-historic Populations."

She walks you through an analysis of two peoples who lived near the Ohio River valley. The farmers, referred to as the "Hardin Village" group in the book, lived in the area about 500 years ago. The hunter-gatherers, who are given the name "Indian Knoll" for the area in which their remains are found, lived in the area 3,000-5,000 years ago. The sites are significant in that each one produces a large number of skeletal remains. For statistical purposes, this makes information derived from the sites more compelling. The agriculture-based Hardin Villagers subsisted mainly on corn, beans, and squash, as is typical of many groups of Native Americans, including the Pima of Mexico and Arizona. The HGs of Indian Knolls subsisted on a mixed foraging diet of meat, wild fruits, fish, and shellfish. The differences in the health of the two people is remarkable:

➤   The HGs show almost no cavities, whereas the farmers showed almost 7 cavities on average per person.
➤   The HGs show significantly less bone malformations consistent with malnutrition. That is—the HG's were much better fed.

➤ The HGs showed a remarkably lower rate of infant mortality relative to the farmers. The most significant difference was between the ages of two and four when malnutrition is particularly damaging to children.

➤ The HGs were, on average, healthier, as evidenced by decreased rates of bone malformations typical of infectious disease.

➤ The HGs on average lived longer than the farmers.

➤ The HGs showed little to no sign of iron, calcium, and protein deficiencies, whereas this was common in the farmers.

The department chair whisks away to make a copy of the chapter for you to take home. (If you'd like to read this chapter in its entirety, visit my website, www.Robbwolf.com, for the links.) You contemplate your next question, while considering the information you were just presented. When she returns, you ask her the only things that come to mind: "Is the situation you showed me typical? Isn't this an exception? Haven't we adapted to eating grains?"

She looks at you sympathetically and contemplates her response for a moment. "Our genetics are nearly identical to those of our early *H. Sapien* ancestors from 100,000–200,000 thousand years ago. We are genetically wired for a lifeway that is all but gone now, and our health reflects this. The change from HG to agriculturalist that I described to you is typical of every transition we have studied. We moved from a nutrient-dense, protein-rich diet that was varied and changed with location and seasons to a diet dependent upon a few starchy crops. These starchy crops provide a fraction the vitamins and minerals found in fruits, vegetables, and lean meats. These "new foods" create a host of other health problems ranging from cancer to autoimmunity to infertility. I have no idea why this is not widely understood by the medical community, but I know for a fact few nutritional science departments offer course work in ancestral diets or the role evolution plays in our health and wellness."

You are now completely sober and not really that happy. This is all feeling very heavy. The department chair seems to detect your disquiet and offers to take you on a tour of the department. She shows you the forensics lab where students are trained in the discovery, identification, collection, and preservation of human remains. You had no idea all the stuff you've see on *CSI* actually had its beginning as an outgrowth of anthropology and the study of ancient humans. We thank the department chair for her time and expertise and wander outside into the warm, Northern California day. We look at each other, and you ask, "Should we go over to the Nutritional Sciences Department?"

"Sure, but you will wish we went and had a few more NorCal margaritas first!"

We make the short walk across campus and enter the hallowed halls of the Department of Nutritional Sciences. Keep in mind, this department exists under the umbrella of the School of Biological Sciences. Just keep that in mind.

We walk into the department and, as luck would have it, several of the faculty are sitting together eating an early afternoon snack of bagels and orange juice. You really need to stay ahead of low blood sugar crashes that happen midday!

We introduce ourselves and mention we have some questions about nutrition and health. The nutrition scientists tell us we have come to the right place, so we launch in with the same question posited to the anthropology professors: What is the most important event in human history?

The nutrition scientists look at each other as if suspecting one of them set this situation up as a joke, but alas this is not a joke. One of them asks us, "What does history have to do with nutrition and health?"

I look knowingly at you and encourage you to take the point on this skirmish. You ask the group, "What about the development of agriculture? Wasn't that important for the health and wellness of our species?"

The nutrition scientists nod slowly, but you can tell they are not comfortable with this situation. Not at all. A gaunt fellow wearing a T-shirt proclaiming, "Tofu: It's What's for Dinner," chimes in.

"Of course this was important. Prior to agriculture people lived short, brutish lives".

Another posits, "Yes, it's hard to catch animals and the "stable" food supply of agriculture allowed the population to expand. Humans developed art and science and medicine."

We both concede the truth of cultural development, but you mention the change in health and wellness the anthropology professors related to us just an hour earlier. You mention the remarkable health of our Paleolithic ancestors as described by the anthropology professors. You mention the difference between the skeletons of agriculturalists versus hunter-gatherers.

The group of nutrition scientists are really not happy now. One quips, "How are we to know what our ancestors ate? This is all conjecture." Another faculty member, who has a body mass index of 32, adds, "Just because our ancestors ate that way does not mean it's healthy. All those people died young, undoubtedly from the meat they ate. Everyone knows meat gives you cancer."

You reply that the anthropology professors related the fact hunter-gatherers appeared to suffer virtually no cancer until they adopted grains, legumes, and dairy. We are met with eye rolling and muttering. This exchange of ideas is quickly coming to a close.

I ask a few more questions: "The Nutritional Sciences Department, it's under the auspices of the School of Biological Sciences, yes?" Everyone nods agreement. "So, really, the nutritional sciences should be looked at as a branch of biology, yes?" More nods of agreement. "What is the foundational, guiding tenet of biology? What idea is used to make sense of the ever-increasing amounts of information in the various branches of biology? What is the idea that ties together *all* of biology?" I'm met with blank looks. "Do you use the concept of evolution via natural selection to guide you as scientists?"

To this, one of the nutrition scientists responds, "Evolution has obvious application to the biological sciences, but it is of limited utility in understanding human beings."

"So, humans are exempt from the laws of biology?" I ask this person.

This creates a little mumbling that winds down to stony silence. These nice people would like to see our backsides. I ask one more question: "What *do* you use to make dietary recommendations?" To this the cheerful nutrition scientist wearing the tofu T-shirt responds, "Oh! We use this!" And he slides me a copy of the USDA "My Pyramid" food guide.

The Rest of the Story

The story above is just that, a story. I've taken significant liberty here, but it has a remarkable thread of truth. I have had this conversation with faculty in the Nutritional Sciences Department (at CSU Chico and elsewhere) that was essentially the same as related in my fable above. The people who push and promote the nutritional guidelines for most of the Westernized world do not believe our hunter-gatherer origins have any bearing on our health. These people *think* they are scientists, yet when their feet are held to the fire, they have no science to stand upon. Physicists have theories such as quantum mechanics and relativity, which they use to answer questions about our world. These theories provide the continuity to evaluate the new information we gather.

Occasionally, our information forces us to reevaluate our models, but we know we are onto something good when we can use our model to make predictions. Physicists would not dream of operating without the models they have, yet the vast majority of people in medicine and the nutritional sciences have no idea where to look for a unified theory of health and wellness. This is due in part to laziness and, literally, a lack of thinking things through. People are spoon-fed ideas that make no sense (fat makes you fat, yet the people who eat more fat, like the French, Spanish and Greeks, are not as fat as we are. We will just call this finding "paradoxical" and move along without thinking). This laziness might be excusable if it was not costing billions of dollars and cutting short hundreds of thousands of lives. I won't even get into the people who are profiteering from your early demise with pharmaceuticals and processed foods.

The point I'd like to make is this: *You are on your own.* You can walk into your doctor's office with horrible blood work, all while eating a low-fat, high-carb diet of "whole grains." You can then shift to an ancestral way of eating that involves lean meats, seafood, seasonal vegetables, and fruit. Walk back into your doctor's office with perfect blood work, yet he will not believe that eating more protein and fat is what fixed your broken blood work. We are working to develop a physician network of doctors educated in evolutionary medicine and the Paleo diet—I just hope we can keep you alive long enough to see one.

Now that we understand a little more about our hunter-gatherer ancestry and the blinders most of medicine and nutritional sciences are wearing, it's time to learn a little science so you can make sense of your Paleo Solution. It won't hurt, and it will likely save or dramatically improve your life.

THREE

◇◇

Knowledge Is Power, But It Will Not Run A Hair Dryer

◇◇

I'm not going to spend a huge amount of time trying to scare you into action, but you might need a little more convincing. You have *questions*. You want to know why cardiovascular disease, cancer, diabetes, autoimmunity, and infertility are on the rise? Why is it that these conditions are largely preventable (they are), yet our government does not tell us how to prevent them? I must admit, these are some pretty good questions, and we have not even gotten to things like, "Does cholesterol cause heart disease?" or "does protein cause kidney damage?"

To answer these questions I need to do a little explaining. I'm not going to spend a chapter on each of these topics, detailing the pathophysiology of each disease, but I need to look at some of the basics. If you want to skip to the "how to" chapters, go for it. As I mentioned before, you do not need to understand any of this to *do* it. But if you skip your homework, if you take this shortcut, you need to do exactly what I tell you, and you don't get to ask *any* questions!

You still with me? Good. However, I have to warn you. The answers to these questions require some of that nerdy "sciency" stuff. While it might be a bit technical, trust me when I tell you that you'll do better once you earn your nutri-geek-decoder ring. If you don't have your sights set on this precious bauble, you can still learn the essence of the science. For the pocket-protector crowd, I have separated some of the tougher material and placed it in the geek-speak sections throughout the text.

All Roads Lead To . . .

Keep in mind, we *can* prevent or reverse cancer, diabetes, neurodegeneration, and infertility (depending upon how far down the path to destruction you may have wandered). You might have noticed many of these diseases occur together. Heart disease *and* depression. Infertility *and* autoimmunity. This is because these seemingly separate diseases share an underlying mechanism: Inflammation. Inflammation is a natural process that we will die without, but we will also die with too much. This is a case of Goldilocks wanting things to be "just right."

I'm going to walk you through the mechanisms behind your Inflammation Apocalypse and hopefully convince you to change your "evil" ways. Then we will get down to fixing y'all's little red wagons!

To understand how food influences inflammation, which is the underlying cause of diabetes, cardiovascular disease, Parkinson's, and Alzheimer's, we need to understand just a little bit about digestion and the hormonal consequences of our food.

I'm going to define a few terms before we get started. We need to understand the players in digestion, starting with what our food is made of (protein, carbohydrate, and fat) and the hormonal signals that are released in response to food (or the lack thereof). Armed with this information, we can begin to understand how food choices today can manifest as either health or disease tomorrow. In addition, we will learn a dizzying array of polysyllabic terms that only a biochemist could love. Please keep hands inside the ride at all times, do not feed croflora.

Digestion: From Your Pie Hole to Your Hoo-Ha in 453 Easy Steps

Proteins

Proteins are what make up our skin, muscle, hair, and nails, to say nothing of neurotransmitters, enzymes, and hormones. Good sources of protein include fish, fowl, meat, eggs, and shellfish. Some well-intentioned but misguided souls will tell you that you can get protein from beans and rice, nuts and seeds. That's true, but these are what I call "third world proteins." They will keep you alive, but they will not make you thrive. This should be clear from the previous chapter that compared hunter-gatherer and agrarian societies.

Proteins are made of molecules called amino acids. Our physiology makes use of twenty-one amino acids, eight of which are "essential." We *must* get them from our food. Think about amino acids and proteins like different building blocks that allow you to construct cool stuff, like giraffes, whales, hormones, and steaks!

Carbohydrates

Technically, carbohydrates include everything from wood to grass to apples to bread. Depending on how you link carbohydrates together, you can have anything from a plate of pasta to a sequoia, but it all starts simply, with what are called "monosaccharides." *Mono*, of course, means "single." *Sacchar* means "sugar." So, monosaccharide literally means "one sugar." The two monosaccharides, or sugars, we will follow most closely are glucose (the main sugar used for energy in our bodies) and fructose (a relative of glucose). Think about fructose like a drunk aunt at a family reunion: She seems nice enough, but wreaks havoc wherever she goes.

Next we have "disaccharides," which means "two sugars." You are all familiar with sucrose (table sugar)—this is a disaccharide of glucose and fructose.

Finally, we have "polysaccharides," which literally means "many sugars." For our jaunt through your digestive tract, we will consider two types of polysaccharides—indigestible carbohydrates, which we commonly refer to as fiber (both soluble and insoluble), and digestible polysaccharides we know as starch. Rice, potatoes, corn, and flour are all examples of polysaccharides/starch. The next time you have a chubby physician or dietician tell you that complex carbs are healthy, ask yourself, *Does it make sense that "many sugars" might be good for me?* Hmmm.

Fats

There are quite a number of fats, and we will consider specific fats in a later chapter, but for now we just need to know that what we commonly refer to as "fat" is called a triglyceride—an alcohol-like molecule called glycerol that is attached to three fatty acids. Think about triglycerides like a molecular party: glycerol brings the "booze," the fatty acids bring the energy and good times!

Hormones: for Digestion and Fun or Can You Hear Me Now?

Now that we know the players (protein, carbohydrate, and fat), let's see how they fit into digestion, hormonal release, and eventually health and disease.

How does your body know it's "hungry"? What does "hunger" really mean? You likely have a much better social life and get out more than I do, so you have never pondered these riveting topics, but since we are here, we might as well ask the important questions—and they *are* important.

Understanding how our body normally regulates hunger will give us insight into the development of obesity, cancer, diabetes, and a number of other nasty problems we would all do well to avoid. Similar to the fuel gauge of an automobile, our sense of hunger tells us when our body is running out of stored energy. But when we eat, we need to know when we have had enough. Hunger lets us know when we are "running on empty" and the sense of satiety tells us when the fu[are full.

All of this information is communicated throughout the body by chemical messengers called hormones. Before you are finished with this book, you will "meet" quite a number of hormones and you will understand a good bit of what they do in critters such as yourself. In simple terms, hormones are messengers that communicate information throughout the body. How we age, burn fat, think, and reproduce are largely controlled by hormones.

Each hormone has a very specific way of interacting with the cells in our bodies. They interact through a molecule called a receptor site. A common analogy for hormones and receptors is the picture of a lock and key. The key would be the hormone, which fits snugly into the specific "lock" (receptor). This analogy is helpful in that it describes accurately the physical interaction of a hormone and receptor based on shape, but it is a bit odd to imagine keys floating about your body.

I like the additional analogy of hormones acting like radio signals and receptors acting like receivers tuned to specific hormones. The combination describes both the physical interaction of the hormone and receptor, but also the fact that information can be transmitted across vast distances by the hormone, which is then received by the receptor site. Hormonal communication in the body controls our levels of body fat, our thinking, our hunger, and just about anything you can think of.

Now let's look at the main hormone players, beginning with insulin.

Insulin is critical in regulating blood sugar, body fat, and aging. To live long, look good, and keep our marbles, we would do well to keep our insulin on the low side by controlling carbs and certain lifestyle factors.

Geek-Speak

Insulin acts as a nutrient-storage hormone that maintains blood glucose levels. In simple terms, insulin puts nutrients into our cells. What we will find, however, is that insulin plays a key role in a staggering number of critical processes completely unrelated to blood sugar management.

Why Is Blood Glucose Important?

So, I mention blood glucose (sugar) levels quite a few times in this book. Why is it important? Well, the red blood cells and certain parts of the brain can run on no other fuel besides glucose. In certain situations like insulin resistance, blood sugar levels can fall and the result can range from dizziness and hunger to unconsciousness and death. So, we should eat lots of carbs then, right? Uh, *no*. As you will see we are better served if we can encourage most of the body to run on fat and just provide enough carbohydrate to meet the needs of these truly glucose-dependent tissues. By reducing the body's total need for carbohydrate, we actually protect ourselves from blood sugar crashes.

Insulin is relevant not only in glucose storage, but also in fat and protein (amino acid) storage. Insulin is released from the beta cells of the pancreas primarily in response to increasing blood levels of glucose and amino acids and plays a significant role in micronutrient storage and conversions. Insulin's primary role as a nutrient sensor (when you ingest food, insulin tells those nutrients where to be stored) greatly influences genetic expression surrounding aging by up or down regulating maintenance and repair at the cellular level. If you are interested in aging, your level of body fat, when or if you will lose your marbles, and whether or not your "reproductive machinery" works, you will want to keep an eye on insulin.

Glucagon helps normalize blood sugar and energy levels between meals by releasing energy from the liver and allowing us to better access our body fat for energy.

Geek-Speak

Glucagon is the counter-hormone to insulin and prompts the release of glucose from the liver, as well as free fatty acids from fat stores, by a process called lipolysis. Glucagon secretion is stimulated by decreased blood glucose levels (hunger), increased blood amino acid levels, and the hormone cholecystokinin (CCK). High levels of insulin, free fatty acids, ketone bodies, or urea in the bloodstream will inhibit glucagon release. Insulin and glucagon play complementary roles of helping us to manage energy levels by storing and releasing nutrients at the right time. Insulin facilitates the passage of nutrients into cells, while glucagon tends to release stored nutrients to be used for energy.

Leptin tells our body how much fuel we have in storage, and when we are "full." If we lose the ability to sense leptin, appetite control is lost.

Geek-Speak

Leptin regulates both appetite and metabolism. Leptin enters the central nervous system where it acts on receptors in the brain that control energy intake and expenditure. Leptin is produced by white adipose tissue (fat cells), as well as the cells lining the wall of the stomach. The leptin produced by the cells in the stomach is responsible for controlling appetite. When Leptin is working correctly, it's very effective at telling us we are "full" after eating a meal. As we will see, when leptin signaling (how a hormone "talks to a receptor") breaks, it is the beginning of problems ranging from cancer to accelerated aging to neurological degeneration.

Ghrelin tells us we are hungry or low on energy. We would like this to be an accurate message, but it is important to note that stress and lack of sleep can alter ghrelin levels and unfavorably increase our sense of hunger.

Geek-Speak

Ghrelin is a hormone that stimulates hunger, increases food intake, and increases fat mass. It is produced by cells in the lining of the stomach, as well as epsilon cells of the pancreas. Ghrelin is also produced in the hypothalamic arcuate nucleus, where it stimulates the secretion of growth hormone. Inadequate sleep is associated with high levels of ghrelin. A little down the road, you will discover just how important sleep is to maintaining a lean, healthy body. Since sleep deprivation increases ghrelin, and since ghrelin increases appetite, this is one of the reasons why sleep disturbance leads to increased food intake.

Adiponectin is another of several satiety hormones. Not only does it tell us when we've had enough food, but it also protects our arteries from oxidative damage.

Geek-Speak

Adiponectin is a protein hormone that is secreted by adipose tissue and has the following effects: decreases gluconeogenesis (the conversion of protein into glucose), increases glucose uptake, and protects from endothelial dysfunction (a common feature of atherosclerosis). Although released by adipose tissue, levels of adiponectin in the bloodstream of adults is inversely correlated with percentage of body fat (folks with low body fat have high adiponectin). Adiponectin is an independent risk factor for metabolic syndrome and plays a role in the suppression of the metabolic derangements that may result in type 2 diabetes, obesity, atherosclerosis, and nonalcoholic fatty liver disease.

Peptide YY (a.k.a. PYY) is yet another hormone trying to tell us when to stop eating. Protein and fat release a lot of PYY and are thus very satisfying. Carbohydrate, by contrast, releases relatively little PYY, which is why your bran muffin and juice breakfast leaves you ravenous in a few hours.

Geek-Speak

PYY is a gut hormone that reduces hunger while simultaneously improving central nervous system sensitivity to leptin. PYY is released by neuroendocrine cells in the ileum and colon in response to feeding. Protein causes greater PYY secretion than fat, which causes greater PYY secretion than carbohydrate. PYY plays a synergistic role with leptin in helping us feel satisfied after a meal.

Cortisol raises blood sugar levels, which can cause fat gain. Although many people don't know this, cortisol release from stress and a lack of sleep factors prominently in body fat gain, leading to that pesky spare tire around the midsection. Cortisol shouldn't be feared, because it is a crucial anti-inflamatory—we just don't want too much of it.

Geek-Speak

Cortisol is often referred to as a "stress hormone," given that it is released in response to stress and anxiety. Cortisol increases blood pressure and acts as an anti-inflammatory by lowering the activity of the immune system. It will trigger the breakdown of muscle mass by converting protein (amino acids) into glucose via gluconeogenesis. Cortisol decreases insulin sensitivity, lowers the rate of bone formation, and causes a loss of collagen in the skin and other connective tissues. The following increase cortisol levels: intense or prolonged physical activity, caffeine, sleep deprivation, stress, subcutaneous fat tissue, and certain contraceptives.

Insulin-like Growth Factor-1 (IGF-1) is another hormone we want "just the right amount" of. It aids in physical recovery, but poor diet can abnormally raise IGF levels, which in turn increases both our likelihood for cancer and our rate of aging.

Geek-Speak

IGF-1 is critical to the growth of children and has an anabolic effect in adults. IGF-1 activates the insulin receptor but generates a response that is only 10 percent of that observed for insulin. Low IGF-1 promotes cell maintenance and stress resistance. IGF-1 levels are highest during pubescent growth spurts. Exercise, stress, and nutrition can affect IGF-1 levels. Increased levels of IGF-1 stimulate both growth and aging.

Now that you have met the players in this digestion/endocrinology orchestra, you likely understand a little about the chemistry of our food and "who" the primary hormones are that we must consider in digestion, health, and disease. Gold star for you. This is a nice start, but we have some more work to do. Next, we need to consider what actually happens to both our food and our hormones during various conditions like fasting and overeating. With this knowledge we will be in a position to understand Type 2 diabetes, various types of cancer, Alzheimer's, Parkinson's, infertility, cardiovascular disease, and osteoporosis.

FOUR

◇◇

Digestion:
Where The Rubber Hits The Road

◇◇

You find the last chapter a bit overwhelming? Do you need an espresso? A hug? Don't worry, this will all make sense soon. To understand how all these different pieces fit together, we need to track a typical meal that contains some protein, carbohydrate, and fat through the digestive process. "From the lips to the hips," as it were. Let's make this a meal of baked salmon (protein), avocado (fat), and fruit salad (carbohydrate). We will track not only the digestive fate of our meal, but also the hormonal effects of:

1. Normal eating
2. No eating at all (fasting)
3. Overeating

We are looking at this because things like type 2 diabetes occur when the normal hormonal signals associated with food (I'm hungry, I'm full. Where's the remote?) get "lost." It is the loss of this hormonal communication that leads to obesity, accelerated aging, many types of cancers, and the other health issues we will consider. Let's get digesting!

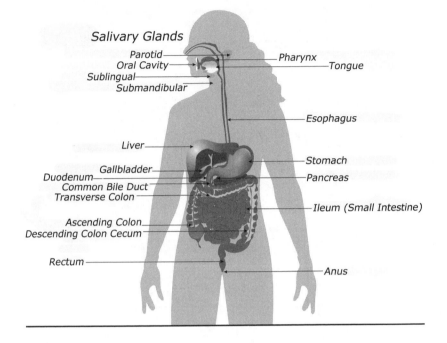

The Mouth: Salivary Glands, Teeth, and Garden Supplies

For simplicity, let's assume we take a bite of our meal that contains all three ingredients—a little salmon, avocado, and fruit salad.

Big picture: From a digestive perspective, the mouth is mainly about the physical breakdown of our food. Chewing breaks large pieces of food into smaller pieces, making it ready for chemical and enzymatic digestion later in the process.

Protein: Our baked salmon is broken down into smaller pieces but remains chemically unchanged.

Carbs: The fruit salad is an interesting mix of monosaccharides (glucose and fructose), disaccharides (sucrose, which is glucose and fructose again), polysaccharides in the form of starch (many glucose molecules connected together, which we can digest), and fiber (which is important for digestive health, but we do not break it down—Unless you are a termite).

Salivary amylase begins the process of breaking down starch in the mouth. This has very little activity due to the relatively short time in the mouth, especially if you are like my wife and take your food down like a boa constrictor.

The sweet taste from the fruit "primes the pump" for the rest of the digestive process. This is an electrochemical communication between the taste buds and the brain, and the rest of the digestive system. As we will see later, this system can be fooled by artificial sweeteners with truly catastrophic effects.

Fat: The avocado is reduced to a paste in the mouth but is chemically unaltered.

The Stomach: Hydrochloric Acid, Pepsin, Parietal Cells, and Ladies' Wear

Big picture: The stomach is an acid environment that plays host to a small amount of protein digestion by the action of acid and the enzyme pepsin. The stomach is really just staging the food for the serious digestion a few stops down the line. Cells that line the stomach sense food and release leptin into the circulation. Leptin passes into the brain, signaling the appetite centers that we are "fed," thus decreasing appetite, while *increasing* our metabolic rate in response to food.

This increase in metabolic rate is manifested mainly as an increase in fat "burning" for energy. The stomach releases several hormones to stimulate downstream digestion. One of these is cholecystokinin (CCK), which is another hormone that sends a satiety ("I'm full") signal to the brain while also stimulating the release of bile salts and pancreatic enzymes in the next step. Although this is still very early in the digestive process, communication with the brain is already occurring that we are "fed." What might happen if this signal is sluggish or absent?

Protein: A small amount of chemical and enzymatic digestion occurs in the stomach. Imagine thousands, perhaps tens of thousands, of amino acids strung together. The digestion in the stomach breaks them down, but the pieces are still large. Our salmon still looks like salmon for the most part.

Carbs: No digestion occurs in the stomach.

Fats: Virtually no fat digestion occurs in the stomach. In the stomach, fat and carbs are just hanging out, drinking coffee, and playing cards to pass the time.

Small Intestines: Pancreatic Enzymes, Bile Salts, and Home Appliances

Big picture: The acidic contents of the stomach (now called chyme) are emptied into the first portion of the small intestine called the duodenum. Bicarbonate is injected into the chyme to change the mixture from an acidic to a basic environment. The enzymes that break down protein, carbohydrate, and fat work best within narrow pH (acid/base) ranges. The stomach is acidic enough to dissolve a penny, but the main digestion, which happens in the small intestine, is an alkaline or "basic" environment. Baking soda is an example of a common base.

As the chyme enters the small intestines, it is mixed with pancreatic enzymes (not surprisingly, from the pancreas!) and bile salts released by the gall bladder. Folks, the real fun is about to begin!

Protein: The proteins, which are now hundreds or thousands of amino acids long, are rapidly reduced to tri- and dipeptides (three- and two- amino acid proteins) by the action of pancreatic enzymes. These small peptides are finally cleaved into single amino acids as the peptides interact with the brush border of the small intestines. The brush border has enzymes that catalyze this reaction of small peptides into free, single amino acids. The free amino acids enter the blood stream and are transported to the liver, and then the rest of the body for use in growth and maintenance.

Carbs: Monosaccharides can enter the blood stream directly, just like amino acids. However, disaccharides like sucrose must be cleaved into monosaccharides at the brush border of the intestines. And polysaccharides such as starch must be broken all the way down into free glucose. The bottom line is that carbohydrates must be reduced to single molecules to be absorbed through the intestinal wall and transported into the circulation. So folks, this is an opportunity to see "complex carbohydrates" for exactly what they are: Lots of sugar. No matter what type of carbohydrate we absorb, it all goes into the system as either glucose or fructose, aka sugar.

Fats: If you recall, when the chyme enters the small intestines from the stomach, pancreatic enzymes and bile salts are mixed into the party. The bile salts are vitally important in the digestion of fats. As I'm sure you are aware, fats and water do not mix, and if we want to digest fat (and yes, we do want that, my fat-phobic-friends), then we need fat to be dissolved in the bile salts. Bile is virtually identical to soap in that it has a piece that likes to associate with water, and another piece that likes to associate with fats. This is why soap is so effective in cleaning dirty dishes.

This process of dissolving the fats in the bile salts is called emulsification. Once emulsified, the pancreatic enzyme lipase* can break apart the fat, which as you learned earlier, is made up of glycerol and fatty acid molecules. With the glycerol and fatty acids free of one another, they can be transported through the intestinal wall, and are then reassembled on the other side.

The fats (triglycerides/TAGs) must be transported to the liver just like protein and carbohydrates, but as I mentioned before, fats and water do not mix well. This problem is solved by packaging the TAGs

---

Lipase is a term derived from the Greek "lipos," which means "fat," and "-ase," which means to cut. Quite literally, it means to "cut the fat." Whenever you see "-ase," you know it's an enzyme that's involved in a reaction. The world is a never-ending source of amusements when you master a few Greek and Latin suffixes. For example, "kattase" means "cut the cat," while teereease means to, well, "cut the cheese."

with special proteins that carry them to the liver. This whole complex is called a chylomicron, and it plays a central role in cholesterol, which we will consider later. Unlike protein and carbohydrates, fats are transported in the lymph vessels first, then once they enter the general circulation, they make their way to the liver or are used by tissues of the body.

My Liver! My Liver!

Detour! Although digestion in the GI tract is not complete, we have learned as much from that as we need to. Everything beyond this point is just poop anyway! We now need to look at the fate of our macronutrients (protein, carbs, and fat) as they interact with the liver.

Big picture: When nutrients are absorbed through the intestinal lining into circulation, the hormone peptide YY (PYY) is released. It is another player in satiety both directly and because it improves leptin sensitivity. Protein releases a relatively large amount of PYY and is therefore very satiating. Fat releases a significant amount, but less than protein, while carbohydrate releases the least PYY. This should give you a hint of how to construct a meal to improve your sense of satiety (Protein + Fat = Where it's at). Also, you might have noticed that we have met several hormones involved in communication between the digestive system and the brain. When things are working properly, we have excellent appetite control and tend to eat just the right amount of food for our activity and maintenance needs. When this communication breaks down, chaos ensues.

The Fed, the Underfed, and the Ugly

The next section is somewhat like a "choose your own adventure" story in that we will look at three alternate endings with our food. A "normal" fed state in which we take in about as many calories as we need (in geek speak that's isocaloric), the fasted state (hypocaloric), and the overfed state (hypercaloric). Keep in mind, we need to understand all this to make sense of how obesity, cancer, and neurodegeneration can happen when our food no longer sends the hormonal signals that keep us slim and healthy.

Normal Feeding

Protein: Really, we are talking amino acids now, as the protein (salmon) that initiated this meal is now broken into individual amino acids. The fate of amino acids can now go one of a few ways. The liver can absorb amino acids and either use them for its own functioning, convert one amino acid into another form (changing one tinker toy into a different kind), or convert that amino acid into sugar via a process called gluconeogenesis (gluco—glucose, neo—new, genesis—birth or creation).

If amino acids are not used in the liver, they are circulated to the body and used to grow new cells, repair damaged cells, grow hair and skin, make hormones, and a host of other functions. The pool of amino acids in our bodies is considered "labile" or flexible, as we can use proteins from our muscles and other tissues in times of scarcity to make glucose via gluconeogenesis. Many doctors and health authorities want you to believe that you'll keel over and die without carbohydrates. Not true—we have several ways of making carbohydrates from proteins and fats. You will understand this process much better before the end of this chapter.

Carbs: Once carbohydrates are broken down into free glucose by the digestive process, the glucose makes its way from the intestines to the liver quite quickly, but its fate is not yet decided. Free glucose causes the release of insulin from the pancreas as it enters the blood stream. Insulin activates GLUT4, one of several glucose transport molecules found in our cell membranes. Under normal circumstances, these transport molecules facilitate blood glucose absorption by the liver. The glucose is then stored as a form of starch called glycogen. This stored glucose is critically important for maintaining blood glucose between meals. The glucose that is not used by the liver passes to the systemic circulation and is used by the brain, red blood cells, and other tissues as a fuel source. A primary example of this is glycogen being stored in the muscles, which can then be used as energy when performing explosive, short activity. If the carbohydrate amount is relatively small, this is the end of the story. However, we still need to consider fructose.

Fructose must be handled by the liver, as none of the other tissues in the body can utilize fructose directly. Fructose is converted to glucose by the liver and then stored as glycogen. If our fructose intake is low and our total calorie intake is not excessive, things are "OK." But keep your eyes open—excessive fructose is a player in the development of obesity, depression, diabetes, and the associated diseases of metabolic derangement.

Fat: Triglycerides/TAGs are transported to the liver in lipid/protein packages called chylomicrons. The chylomicron can drop off TAGs at the liver or it can carry the TAGs around the body to be dropped off at muscle, organs, or fat cells to be used as fuel. Once a chylomicron has dropped off most of its TAGs, it will make its way back to the liver and be reused in the important cholesterol story, which we will cover in just a bit.

Fasted State

Big picture: The fasted state can mean going completely without food for a period of time or simply a reduced calorie level relative to energy expenditure. As we will see, how our body responds to a calorie deficit is largely dependent on our hormonal state. It may seem odd to consider fasting when we are talking about eating food, but a significant breakdown occurs in the overfed state in which parts of our body "think" it is starving. It's ugly, and we need to understand the mechanisms of fasting to understand how overeating goes so terribly wrong.

Protein: Although protein is critical as a structural element and in maintaining fluid balance with proteins in our blood called albumin, proteins are also fairly expendable. Your body is more concerned about avoiding a blood sugar crash than it is about maintaining muscle mass. That's why during fasting we tend to convert large amounts of amino acids into glucose, which is stored in the liver as glycogen and then released to maintain blood glucose levels. In other words, in a fasted state, your hard-earned muscles might be converted into glucose. As we will see, hormone status and the presence of ketones (you'll meet them in a bit, I promise) can change how much protein we convert to glucose. This is really important if our fast is unintentional and we are facing a long period of starvation.

Carbs: In the fasted state, virtually all dietary carbohydrate is initially sequestered in the liver. Although the muscles and organs like glucose just fine as a fuel, there are other tissues like red blood cells and certain parts of the brain that can run on nothing but glucose. For this reason, the body becomes quite stingy with how it spends its glucose. The adaptable tissues shift to fat and ketone metabolism, saving the glucose for the vital tissues.

Fats: During fasting, the body uses *stored* body fat as a fuel. As the body shifts to fat as a primary fuel source, a by-product of fat metabolism begins to accumulate: ketones. Now, ketosis is *not* a reason for panic! Your doctor and dietician should not confuse ketosis with ketoacidosis (a potentially life-threatening metabolic state). These two states are as different as night and day, and I'll pay good money to hear a doctor or dietician accurately describe the biological distinctions, as most cannot.

The metabolic state of ketosis is normal and almost as old as time. Ketones are like small pieces of fat that are water soluble, and given a few days or weeks, most of our tissues can shift their metabolism to burn ketones. Interestingly, many tissues such as the heart, kidneys, and intestines function *better* on ketones than on glucose.

A metabolic shift to ketosis solves two very important problems:

1. It protects scarce blood glucose by shifting as much of our metabolic machinery as possible to a nearly limitless fuel supply. We have a day or two of liver glycogen, but even if we are relatively lean, we have literally months of stored body fat. A shift to ketosis saves scarce glycogen to be used to maintain minimal blood glucose levels.

2. Ketosis halts gluconeogenesis. The by-products of ketosis block the conversion of amino acids into glucose. This spares muscle mass that would be very valuable in a state of prolonged starvation. In addition to

Geek Rant

Now, this may sound like heresy, but there are no "essential carbohydrates." Our bodies can make all the carbohydrates it needs from protein and fat. Although glucose is critical for many of our tissues, the redundant mechanisms in our bodies for producing glucose indicate it was a fuel that was transient in our past. We are *not* genetically wired for a 50 percent carbohydrate, bran muffin diet, despite what the USDA, AMA, and FDA have to say on the topic. Capisce?

With that clear in your mind, we need to look at one more piece to this puzzle, the "overfed state." This will help us make sense of how eating too much of the wrong food can cause serious problems.

blocking gluconeogenesis from amino acids, ketosis provides a sneaky, alternative way to make glucose using the glycerol backbone of fats. All in all, it's a very efficient system for protecting blood glucose and muscle mass under the stress of starvation.

Overfed State

Big picture: Overfeeding is a problem. I know, shocking, right? Well, here's the thing: our physiology is actually wired to exist at a caloric excess. Goofy dieticians and some "nutritional scientists" will tell you we need to maintain a caloric "balance" to remain slim and healthy. This is baloney. Figuring out a caloric balance is virtually impossible if it's left up to "us." Metabolic studies have shown an enormous variance between people and how they handle calories. One person can overeat several hundred calories every day for years and never gain a kilo. Other people seem to gain weight by *looking* at food. What gives? What's the difference? Hormones and the signals associated with hormones.

It should not come as a surprise that our bodies have complex sensors that tell us not only if our blood glucose is high or low, but also how much total energy we have in storage. Leptin, which tells the brain we are "full," is not only released in response to food, but it is also released from our body fat. This should make sense on a mechanistic level: A relatively large amount of fat will release a relatively large amount of leptin, which sends the signal "I'm full, no need for more food." Conversely, if we are getting very lean and our energy reserves become low, our leptin signal will be low and we experience hunger.

What does all this have to do with overfeeding, health, and disease? As I was saying before, we are wired to live at a caloric excess. Certain foods affect our sense of satiety and the ultimate fate of our food in very different ways. Think about the difference between the satiety signals produced by protein (very satiating) and carbohydrate (in many people low satiety actually acts as an appetite stimulant). What if we are overfed, but for some reason our brain no longer "hears" the "I'm full" signal from the leptin? What if, despite significant overfeeding, we still think we are hungry? That situation creates one hell of a problem, as you will see.

Protein: In the initial stages of protein overfeeding things run as you might expect: Some amino acids are used for structural repair, but any amino acids beyond this are converted to glucose via gluconeogenesis, or burned directly as a fuel. Protein can add to overall caloric excess, but as a stand-alone item, it is virtually impossible to overeat protein due to the potent satiety signal sent to the brain. Part of the reason for this signal is due to a maximal ability of the liver to process protein set at 30–35 percent of total calories. Protein consumption beyond this point for extended periods of time results in a condition called "rabbit starvation," so named by early pioneers of the American West who would succumb to a disease characterized by muscle wasting, lethargy, diarrhea, and eventually death if one relied too heavily on lean game animals such as rabbits. We will take advantage of the satiating effects of protein to help us remain lean and strong, while rounding out our meals with nutritious fruits, vegetables, and good fats to avoid the potential of too much protein.

Carbs: This next piece is going to be longish but wickedly important. Drink some espresso, stick your head out the window, and yell "I've got to get my head back in the game!"

So, you are now familiar with the fate of glucose (and fructose) as it enters the body and is stored as glycogen in either the muscles or liver. What we have not considered is what happens if liver glycogen is completely full but there is still excess free glucose in circulation (high blood glucose levels). Once liver glycogen is full, excess carbohydrates are converted to fat in the form of a short-chain saturated fat called palmitic acid. This palmitic acid (PA) is stitched to a glycerol molecule and packaged with proteins and cholesterol, and the resultant molecule is called a VLDL (very low-density lipoprotein). This PA-rich VLDL molecule is released from the liver and heads out to the body so the fat may be used as a fuel or get stored on our fannies.

DEFCON 1

Although VLDL's move all about the body, one location they interact with is the brain. PA has a very potent effect on our metabolism and our hormonal environment in that it *decreases* our sensitivity to leptin. When the brain, specifically the hypothalamus (the area of the brain responsible for energy regulation), becomes leptin resistant, the satiety signal that is normally sensed from ingested food is lost. We remain hungry, despite elevated blood glucose levels, and continue to eat beyond our needs. We develop a "sweet tooth" because we cannot sense the normal signal sent by leptin that we are "full." Keep in mind, this Palmitic acid (PA) that causes the leptin resistance in the brain leads to our inability to feel full, and is *made from excess dietary carbohydrate.*

DEFCON 2

This process happens in waves. Like the ocean eroding a sand castle, our insulin sensitivity is degraded and we lose the ability to respond properly to the signal. The liver becomes insulin resistant and blood glucose levels drive higher and higher. Insulin sensitivity in our muscle tissue is lost when they can physically store no more glycogen. The gene expression for the GLUT4 transport molecule is down-regulated because the muscles are literally drowning in glucose. This drives blood sugar higher, which drives insulin higher. Eventually, even the fat cells become resistant to insulin. Things are about to get bad rather quickly.

DEFCON 3

Once systemic, full-body, insulin resistance occurs, inhibitory systems in the liver are overwhelmed and blood glucose is converted into fats and VLDLs at such a high rate that fat cannot escape into circulation, and it begins to accumulate in the liver. This is the beginning of non-alcoholic fatty liver disease. The wheels are seriously falling off the wagon by this point, as is evidenced by the next malfunction that occurs: Despite the fact the liver (in fact, the whole body) is swimming in glucose, the liver is insulin resistant and certain cells perceive the "lack of insulin" as low blood sugar. Your body does *not* like low blood sugar. Low blood sugar can kill you, so your body brings the stress hormone cortisol to the "rescue," and it's like throwing gasoline on a fire.

China Syndrome: Full System Meltdown

Cortisol is released to combat the perceived low blood glucose levels with *gluconeogenesis*. Yes, despite high levels of blood glucose from excess carbohydrate, the body now makes *more glucose* by cannibalizing its own tissues. In this case, muscle and organs are "burned" to make more glucose. Keep in mind, the muscles are a primary site of dealing with elevated blood glucose in the first place! So, not only is the situation made worse by adding more glucose to the blood from gluconeogenesis, we have *less* muscle with which to dispose of all that glucose.

This is why type 2 diabetes and insulin resistance is effectively a wasting disease of the muscles, all the while the fat cells experience record growth. Because of the high insulin, blood sugar, and triglycerides, a significant portion of the fat is stored in the abdominal region. This is the telltale sign of insulin resistance: fat stored at the waistline, creating the very sexy "Apple Shape." We have now set the stage for chronically elevated insulin levels and all the fun that brings: Increased rates of cancer, accelerated aging, and neurodegenerative diseases such as Parkinson's and Alzheimer's, obesity and, ultimately, type 2 diabetes, which is characterized by insulin resistance and chronically elevated blood glucose levels.

AGEs: Yes, It Gets Worse!

Although glucose is a critically important fuel for the body, it is also a toxic substance. Sugars have a nasty habit of reacting with proteins in our bodies. These complexes become oxidized and form "advanced glycation end products" (AGEs). They damage proteins, enzymes, DNA, and hormonal receptor sites on the surface of our cells. AGEs are a major cause of the symptoms we take to be normal aging.

When we look at the pathology of several diseases, we will see that they have AGEs as a major causative factor. Our bodies DO produce enzymes to undo AGEs, but they can only undo a certain amount of damage. If our diet is too heavy in carbohydrate, the damage accumulates faster than we can fix it. Some of the worst damage happens in the pancreatic beta cells, which have already taken a beating from overproduction of insulin. The additional oxidative stress can kill the beta cells and, unlike the liver, once these cells are gone, that's it. This situation produces a hybrid form of diabetes characterized by not only insulin resistance, but also an eventual inability to produce insulin. People in this situation look like both a type 1 and type 2 diabetic.

The other effect in the insulin management story is damage directly to the GLUT4 molecules on our cell membranes caused by AGEs and oxidative damage. This further impairs the ability of muscles to absorb and store glucose.

The take-home of AGEs:
1. They accelerate your aging.
2. They damage already precarious insulin and leptin receptors, worsening insulin resistance.
3. They are key players in several degenerative diseases.

I know this is some heavy, complex material. In the next chapter we'll look at an analogy to make some sense of all this. Remember, if you understand how these diseases manifest, you can take appropriate steps to avoid some nasty characters like cancer, diabetes, cardiovascular disease, and premature aging.

Fructose Side Show

Sorry, I need to take a little detour to the insanity of the fructose story. Have you seen the commercials where high-fructose corn syrup is described as "healthy" because chemically it's almost identical to table sugar (sucrose)? The irony is so thick you'd think it was a *Daily Show* parody (It's just as healthy as *sugar!*), but it's just another public relations attempt on the part of agribusiness to sell us an early grave.

Fructose preferentially fills liver glycogen. That means fructose accelerates the process described above in which liver function is destroyed due to carbohydrate overfeeding. This happens directly because the liver is the only tissue that can handle fructose, but it also happens indirectly because eating fructose *increases* the amount of glucose the liver absorbs. Fructose up-regulates the glucose transport molecules in the liver, making the liver "hungry" for sugar. This leads to increased Palmitic Acid production, which leads to leptin resistance. Oh, yeah, since we were talking about AGEs, fructose is seven times more reactive than glucose in forming AGEs. Funny, they do not mention that fact in all the "high-fructose corn syrup is good for you" commercials!

It's the damndest thing—the United States is in a health care crisis, the economy is shaky, and the government subsidizes the production of corn, making high-fructose corn syrup cheaper than dirt. Processed food manufacturers make crap foods that are making us sick, diabetic, and dead too early. The government subsidizes the development of statins and a host of drugs to manage the diseases that are a direct outgrowth of the processed foods they are subsidizing! A hell of a racket, am I right?

OK, back to our regular program:

FIVE

<><><><><><><><><><><><><><><><><><><><><><><><><><><><><>

Resistance Is Futile:
"What We Have Here Is Failure to Communicate"

<><><><><><><><><><><><><><><><><><><><><><><><><><><><><>

Think about yourself as a remarkably complex machine for a moment. What if one of the key control elements in your existence were to malfunction? What if the primary information messenger that determines how long you will live, if you are fertile, if you develop cancer, senility, and a host of diseases—what if that signal became lost in the shuffle? What if parts of you could not hear the signal at all and other parts of you were deafened by the noise of too much "signal"? What if we called that critical signal insulin? Or leptin?

This may seem esoteric, but I guarantee you have experienced something like this at one time. Consider a time when you walked into a room that had a *very* strong odor like perfume or cologne. Now, what happens to your ability to sense that perfume or cologne after ten to fifteen minutes of being in the room? It's much less, right? How about an hour later? You likely cannot even smell the perfume at this point. What has happened is the olfactory nerves in your nose have down-regulated the receptors for that perfume. If you stepped outside for a breath of fresh air and then returned to the room, you would be able to sense the perfume again. Although a simplistic analogy, this is quite similar to the down-regulation that happens when our bodies are subjected to abnormally elevated levels of hormones such as leptin and insulin.

The situation with hormones is far more complex than perfume because there are different mechanisms that can increase or decrease our ability to sense various hormones. For example, we will see how cortisol decreases our ability to sense insulin, while exercise increases our ability to sense insulin, so long as we do not do so much exercise that we release cortisol and damage our insulin sensitivity! That complexity considered, the perfume analogy is still instructive. The take-home point is that a loss of hormonal sensitivity, in this case for insulin or leptin, can lead to chronically elevated insulin levels and a host of health problems. As you will see, controlling these hormones is critical to losing fat, improving athletic performance, avoiding cancer, preventing neurodegeneration, maintaining fertility, slowing aging, and sidestepping the ravages of Inflammation Gone Wild.

Requiem for a Dream

If you have followed what I have written thus far and understand how we can become insulin resistant, the solution should be pretty obvious: control carbohydrate levels and other lifestyle factors influencing insulin and leptin sensitivity. Unfortunately, the medical response to this problem has been dietary and pharmaceutical interventions that generally *raise* insulin levels. It would be a joke if it was not so tragic.

We will now look at a few conditions that are particularly sensitive to the effects of insulin resistance, specifically cardiovascular disease, cancer, and osteoporosis. Keep in mind, inflammation is the cause of virtually everything that ails us—we are simply considering certain diseases that are heavily influenced by insulin, which itself influences or modifies inflammation. This is laying the foundation for understanding how your Paleo Solution will help you to avoid cancer, diabetes, cardiovascular disease, and a host of other ills. If you haven't noticed, we are still looking at the "whys" behind all these problems: Soon we will look specifically at how to fix or prevent them.

Cholesterol

What we generally refer to as "cholesterol" is actually a mix of proteins, TAGs (fatty acids and glycerol), and the actual molecule, cholesterol. We have met one of these players already in the form of VLDL, which is produced in the liver in response to carbohydrate feedings. The other players we will consider are LDL (low-density lipoprotein) and HDL (high-density lipoprotein). VLDL and LDL carry TAGs and cholesterol from the liver to the rest of the body to be used for fuel and the structural elements of cells. HDL has the opposite role and carries lipids and cholesterol from the peripheral body back to the liver for reprocessing. Think about this as a conveyor system moving substances around the body.

The amount of LDLs in a person's blood has shown some correlation to the likelihood of developing cardiovascular disease, but the association is far from perfect. There are people with "low" blood cholesterol with advanced atherosclerosis (deposits of fats and blood cells that narrow and eventually can block arteries) and there are people with high LDL with no atherosclerosis or cardiovascular disease. What we now know is LDLs come in several varieties, some of which are far more problematic than others.

The variety we would "like" to have is a large, puffy flavor of LDL that floats benignly through the blood stream, dropping its contents at cells that require TAGs or cholesterol. This large, puffy, nonreactive LDL is born in the liver from a backbone of TAGs and structural proteins.

The LDL form we would do well to avoid is a small, dense variety that has a nasty tendency to get stuck in the surface of the epithelial cells lining our arteries. When this happens, our immune system attacks what appears to be a foreign invader and the process damages the arterial lining. Like fiddling with a missing tooth, once these blood vessels are damaged, our immune system will not leave the area alone and the process tends to feed-forward, getting worse and worse.

The small, dense, reactive LDLs are born from the VLDL that is the product of *high-carbohydrate intake*. Although the types of dietary fats we consume do influence these LDLs to a small degree, the main influence is the amount and types of *dietary carbohydrate*. In case you missed that, a high-carbohydrate diet, like the one your doctor, the government, and the pharmaceutical companies endorse, is the type of diet that makes small, dense reactive LDL particles. Good to know these people are fighting *for* your health! Imagine if they were really trying to kill you.

Cardiovascular Disease

The processes that underlies stroke and heart attack involves two main features: Damage to the endothelium (the sensitive layer of cells that line the interior of our veins and arteries) and increased thrombic potential (the likelihood of making a blood clot). The endothelium has an important job of helping to control blood pressure by sensing blood volume and sending signals to the brain to contract or relax the vascular bed to help optimize blood pressure. The endothelium is also important in transporting nutrients throughout the body. All of the protein, carbohydrate, and fat we transport throughout the body for energy must pass through the endothelium on the way to our tissues such as the heart, brain, and muscles.

If our system is inflamed, the likelihood of the endothelium becoming damaged and irritated while transporting nutrients through its membrane is greatly increased. If an area is damaged, the immune system can overreact (especially if we are inflamed, see how all this starts fitting together?) and cause a scar or lesion in the endothelium. This sets the stage for a narrowing of the vessel, which can reduce the flow of oxygen-rich blood to vital organs such as the heart and brain.

This situation is bad, but the literal death blow can come from a blood clot that is caused by our increased levels of inflammation. Our modern diet conspires against us by not only damaging the vessels that carry our life's blood, but also increasing the potential for developing a blood clot, which can cause a life-ending heart attack or stroke. High insulin levels make the whole inflammatory process worse. As do imbalances in essential fats, food intolerances and, as we will learn in the Lifestyle chapter, stress and lack of sleep.

High Blood Pressure

As if effects of elevated insulin on cholesterol were not bad enough, we add insult to injury when blood pressure increases in response to elevated insulin levels. When blood insulin levels increase, we make more of a hormone called aldosterone. Aldosterone causes our kidneys to retain sodium. In biology classes there is a common saying "water follows salt." If we retain sodium, we retain water. And when we retain water, the pressure increases in our arteries and veins, making it easier for them to become damaged. Turbulent flow irritates the vascular beds and causes them to thicken. This thickening, combined with arterial plaques, can narrow the vital arteries to our heart, brain, and other organs. If we want things to get *really* bad, we just need a little calcium. Luckily, that stuff stays locked away in the bones. . . . or does it?

Osteoporosis Link to Cardiovascular Disease (CVD)

Most people with CVD also have some degree of osteoporosis. The common feature is hyperinsulinism (elevated insulin levels). When our insulin levels increase, we tend to secrete the stress hormone cortisol, and the combination of cortisol and insulin work together to leach the mineral calcium from our bones. You may think of your bones as static and unchanging, but they are alive and change based on the demands placed upon them and the hormonal environment we present them.

We are told that we (particularly women) lose bone density as we age. This is only true if we present a hormonal environment that leaches calcium from our system. The Paleo Solution is the perfect antidote for this situation, as it provides adequate minerals to build bones, the proper acid/base balance to spare calcium, and it heals the gut, allowing us to absorb minerals and cofactors critical to bone health such as vitamin D (we will look at all these topics in subsequent chapters).

Now, this whole mess might not be that compelling until you realize that the bone you lost from your skeleton due to high insulin levels goes somewhere. Some of it gets excreted out of your body in the urine. However, some of that calcium just moves to a new place in your body: the lining of your arteries. This is the calcified plaque that lines your arteries and veins in CVD.

The solution we are given for CVD is a high-carb, low-fat diet that keeps insulin levels high. The solution for the osteoporosis is to take a calcium supplement. Little does our doctor know that calcium supplementation is known to be a precipitating factor in blood clots that lead to stroke and heart attack. Oops! Hey, it's just your life folks!

A Paleo diet supplies more magnesium than calcium, which is what our bodies have adapted to over millions of years. High magnesium intake relaxes constricted arteries, lowering blood pressure, while providing the right building materials to keep your bones strong throughout your life, all while keeping your arteries clear and healthy. We will look at common questions and counterpoints to the Paleo diet later in the book, but the calcium/bone health issue is one of the first to be raised by most health "experts." I hope you see that a high-carb, low-fat diet is not the route to keeping your heart, or your bones, strong and healthy.

Insulin, Cancer, and Fertility

It's difficult to find a disease that is not affected by hyperinsulinism. All you need to do is use an Internet search engine, type in your disease of interest, and then add the term "hyperinsulinsim." Even susceptibility to infectious disease is modified by our insulin status, so it is a remarkably broad ranging problem.

I cannot devote a chapter to every nuance of hyperinsulinsim. I know, it's a bummer, but I do need to hit some of the biggies. Just keep in mind, this is a small sampling and by no means a complete accounting of the problems caused by excessive inflammation born of our modern lifestyle.

Cancer: The Short Course

In simple terms, cancer is a wee-bit of "us" that has lost its way. Normally our tissues grow, repair, and eventually die. Although the mechanisms for various types of cancer differ in specific ways, we can make a few generalities:

1. **DNA damage.** The DNA we have in every cell is the blueprint for everything our bodies make. Complex regulatory mechanisms control if we make a certain protein or if a cell replicates. Let's say you start working out and develop some calluses on your hands. The irritation to the skin on your hands causes an increased rate of growth of the skin cells in your hand, producing a layer of thicker skin called a callus. Now, this is all well and good, but whenever a cell replicates (grows), the potential exists for an error to occur when those cells copy the

DNA. The DNA can be hit by radiation or a simple replication error can occur, but the thing to keep in mind is the more replication (growth) that occurs, the higher the likelihood for an error. Imagine if you had to copy the contents of this book. Then, copy the copy and so on. The greater the number of copies, the higher the likelihood of problems.

2. **Loss of growth control.** Our cells have a mechanism called apoptosis that protects us from cancer. If a cell or tissue should become abnormal and start growing in an uncontrolled manner, a safety mechanism, apoptosis, causes the abnormal cell to die.

An Error in Our Ways, a Loss of Control

Many types of cancer, including breast, colon, prostate, and various types of brain tumors share a common mechanism related to hyperinsulinism and it looks like this:

Insulin is a growth promoter of various tissues. So, it causes increased rates of growth all by itself. Insulin also increases the potent growth promoter insulin-like Growth Factor (IGF), while also increasing the levels of androgens such as testosterone and estrogen by *decreasing* a control protein called sex hormone binding protein (SHBP). The net effect is radically increased rates of growth of many tissues. This increases the likelihood of some kind of a DNA error that could cause uncontrolled growth (cancer). This is not an ideal situation, but thankfully the process of apoptosis *normally* saves us from cells that have become precancerous. Well, until elevated insulin levels derail the process of apoptosis. When insulin levels are chronically elevated, a key regulator of apoptosis, retinoic acid (a derivative of vitamin A) is decreased. The stage is now set for abnormal levels of growth, which increases the likelihood of DNA errors that lead to cancer. Our safety net, apoptosis, has also been taken off-line. Our total likelihood of developing cancer has increased dramatically due to hyperinsulinism.

How is that bagel and "whole wheat bread" looking now?

Even if this situation does not cause cancer, it can cause a host of other problems. Prostate enlargement, polycystic ovarian syndrome (PCOS), uterine fibroids, nearsightedness (myopia), fibrocystic breast disease, infertility (both male and female), alopecia (hair loss), and a host of other problems. It goes without saying that normalizing your insulin sensitivity (and other parameters of inflammation) can markedly improve these and many other problems. For folks trying to conceive, you need to really take this stuff seriously.

Ok, I suspect you are about to slip into the fetal position if we talk about insulin much more! Let's take a break from insulin for a little while, but do keep its effects in mind while we look at the other primary sources of inflammation:

⅄ How certain foods damage our digestion.
⅄ How an imbalance of fats alters how we respond to inflammation.
⅄ How the hormone cortisol is wreaking havoc with our health.

Once we are familiar with these issues, we will understand how they synergistically combine in diseases such as cancer, autoimmunity, diabetes, and infertility. Then, we will finally get down to fixing these problems or, even better, preventing them in the first place.

SIX

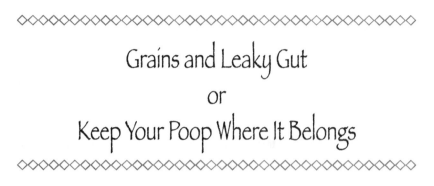

Grains and Leaky Gut

or

Keep Your Poop Where It Belongs

Below I describe several people who at first glance appear different, but in fact they all share some common bonds. They had significant health issues with no apparent cause or solution and assumed they had no treatment options, as their doctors were stumped and could offer few solutions. Fortunately for these folks, they tried a simple experiment and discovered health and healing was only a meal away.

For you, this chapter may represent the "missing link" in your quest for improved performance, health, and longevity. Although our government recommends that you consume grains by the bushel, you will soon see this has everything to do with propping up a pathological oil-agriculture-pharmaceutical complex and nothing to do with your health. I think you will find these stories both interesting and eerily familiar.

Alex, Age Five

I first learned of Alex from my friend Kelly. She related a story of a little boy who was very sick, underweight, and suffering from constant digestive problems. If you like kids and other small, scurrying critters, Alex's features and symptoms were literally heartbreaking. He had painfully skinny arms and legs, attached seemingly at random to a torso dominated by a prominently distended belly. At night Alex thrashed and turned in his bed, wracked by diffuse pain in his arms, legs and, especially, his belly. Alex had severe lethargy and a "failure to thrive." His doctors ran extensive tests but found nothing conclusive. They recommended a bland diet of toast, rice puddings, and yogurt, but with no benefit to the little guy.

Kelly contacted me on behalf of the family and asked if I had any ideas that might help Alex. I made a few specific recommendations, which the parents enacted immediately. Within ten days, Alex's perpetually distended belly was flat and normal. He gained six pounds in a little over two weeks and was noticeably more muscular in the arms and legs. His sleep shifted from the thrashing, restless bouts that left him listless and tired, to the sleep all kids should have: restful, unbroken, and filled with dreams. Alex's energy improved to such a degree that the other kids and parents could hardly imagine he was the same kid. He was healthy and happy, all because of a simple adjustment he and his family made to his eating.

Sally, Age Sixty-One

Sally was referred to us by her family physician. Sally's doctor had worked with her on a variety of issues: low thyroid, osteoporosis, gall bladder problems, depression, and high blood pressure. It was an impressive and ever-growing list of ailments that both Sally and her doctor attributed to "normal" aging. Her doc was pretty forward thinking, however, in that she recommended that Sally perform "weight bearing exercise" to help slow the progression of the osteoporosis and muscle wasting that been accelerating in the past four to five years.

When this recommendation brought Sally to us, she was a bit reluctant to get started with a strength-training program and was *very* reluctant to modify or change her nutrition. We were gentle but persistent.

Our recommendations focused on specific changes to her nutrition and lifestyle. Within two months Sally was off her thyroid medications, her gall bladder issues were gone, she was four pants sizes smaller, while her symptoms of depression had disappeared. After six months of training with us and following our nutrition recommendations, it was discovered that she was no longer osteoporotic.

Of all the improvements, Sally's doctor was most impressed with the increased bone density. She asked Sally what she had modified to affect this change. When Sally told her doctor how she had changed her nutrition, her doctor pondered things for a moment, then said, "Well, it must be something else! Food can't do all that."

Jorge, Age Forty

Jorge started working with us primarily to lose weight. At five feet nine inches and 325 pounds, Jorge was heading down a path of significant illness stemming from type 2 diabetes and obesity. Compounding Jorge's situation was a condition neither he nor his doctors could figure out. Nearly every time Jorge ate, he would break out in a rash and his tongue would swell. Like *really* swell. Jorge had to keep an epi-pen on his person at all times, similar to someone who has a severe allergy to bee stings or peanuts.

Jorge is a practicing attorney and several times a week he would dash out of the courtroom on a mad trip to the emergency room, where he would receive antihistamines to bring his tongue swelling under control. His doctors were (again) stumped. His blood work did not show a specific allergy, nor did he appear to have a full-blown autoimmune disease. Certain immune cells were obviously overactive, but in an atypical fashion that left the allergists and rheumatologists scratching their heads.

We recommended a nutritional change for Jorge, which he fought tooth and nail. God has never made a person more appropriate to be an argumentative lawyer! Part begging, part threatening, we finally won Jorge over and told him, "Just do this for a month. If it does not work, what have you lost? If it does work, what will you have gained?"

Jorge gave things a shot and his tongue swelling disappeared. Now a year later, Jorge is down to 255 pounds and making headway toward his goal of a lean, strong 225 pounds. Thankfully, Jorge now argues *for* us instead of *against* us! Not to beat up on the physicians too much, but when Jorge told his docs what he changed, they too did not believe the cause and effect staring them straight in the face.

So, What the Frack Did We Do?

It will come as a surprise for most people that the underlying cause of all the issues described above, in these very different people, was the same thing—a common component in nearly everyone's diet. Something medicine is only now discovering to be dangerous and unhealthy, despite its prominent role in our food supply. Gluten.

Gluten is a protein found in wheat, rye oats, and barley. Other grains such as corn and rice have similar, but less problematic proteins (we will talk about that later). Just let that soak in for a minute. The usual response is BS! Grains are healthy! The government says so! I love bread and cookies!

OK Buttercup, calm down, I get it. Bread, pasta, and cookies *are* yummy. They are also likely killing you. The other sections of this book I'm willing to give you a "pass" on understanding the technical points. Most people kinda get the insulin/high-carb issue. People are slowly realizing there are "good fats." So, I'll not hold you responsible for *that* material. However, I *insist* you read this grain issue, ponder it, and then *do* what I recommend. Why? Because left to your own devices you will argue and bellyache. Then you will generate an impressive but ultimately inaccurate list of counterarguments and excuses based on emotions, fear, and governmental inaccuracies. Then we have the teensy issue that you are likely more addicted to junk foods than a crackhead to his rock.

Let me be completely clear on this: Your understanding of this situation is clouded by failed governmental policy, the industrial food complex, and *your addiction* to these foods. You may think this is caca-de-torro*, but I'm going to prove you wrong and hopefully save your life in the process. I am not trying to be a jerk, but if you have any of the plethora of health issues for which gluten is a causative factor, the clock is ticking.

We are going to learn the whole story about gluten, grains, and their roles in disease. I'll then give you quantifiable measures for determining how much healthier you are without them. Then it's all up to you. If you want to be healthy,

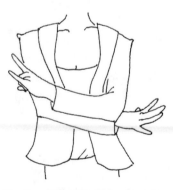

*For the readers who lack a deep steeping in Spanish, here is the same statement in American sign language.

you will find some level of compliance that works for you. If not, we gave it our best shot.

One Cannot Live on Bread at All

We have all seen pictures or videos of smokers dying from lung cancer yet still smoking through tracheotomy holes in their throats. Amazing, right? How can people *do* that? Well, gluten consumption is on par with a pack-a-day smoking habit. And, it's addictive. By the end of this chapter you will understand the health implications. I will try to motivate you to change your ways, but ultimately it's up to you.

Like most things, we need to start at the beginning if we want to understand the whole (grain?) story, so put down that cookie—I'm trying to save your life! First we need to understand what makes up grains so we can understand what grains do to our health and wellness.

Grains Anatomy

When I say "grain," I am talking about one of many domesticated grasses in the *gramineae* family. This includes staples such as wheat, rye, oats, barley, millet, rice, and sorghum. These plants are derivatives or descendants from wild grasses that have been managed and bred for 2,000–5,000 years. All grains have the following anatomy:

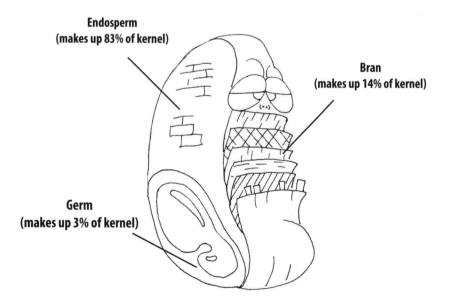

Endosperm
(makes up 83% of kernel)

Bran
(makes up 14% of kernel)

Germ
(makes up 3% of kernel)

Bran

The bran is the outer covering of a whole, unprocessed grain. It contains vitamins, minerals, and a host of proteins and antinutrients designed to prevent the predation, or eating, of the grain. When you see brown rice, the bran is the flakey outer covering of the rice.

Endosperm

The endosperm is mainly starch with a bit of protein. This is the energy supply of a growing grain embryo. When you see white rice, this is the endosperm with bran and germ removed.

Germ

The germ is the actual reproductive portion of the grain. This is where the embryo resides.

In the wild, the cereal grain is distributed by the wind, and when conditions are right, the germ (embryo) begins the process of growth using the endosperm for energy. It may come as a surprise, but plants are not benign, altruistic organisms just waiting to send their next generation of young into our mouths in the form of sushi rice or French bread. Grains, like all critters on this planet, face the challenge of surviving long enough to reproduce. This is particularly problematic for grains in that their most nutrient-dense portion (the part we eat) happens to be the reproductive structure.

Hey Robb, I appreciate your concern, but my dietician told me Oats are gluten free, so no need to worry about my morning bowl of oatmeal? Yep, I love oatmeal too, but it contains similar proteins to gluten. Cereal grains tend to have proteins that are high in the amino acid proline. These prolamines (proline rich proteins) are tough to digest, and thus remain intact despite the best efforts of the digestive process to break them down. The result is gut irritation, increased systemic inflammation, and the potential for autoimmune disease.

Corn has a similar prolamine called zein. Now you can heed or disregard this information as you please, but grains are a significant problem for most people. Upon removal of these grains (as you will learn about in the implementation chapter), you will notice that you feel better. With reintroduction of grains…well, you feel worse. Keep in mind this inflammation is also a factor in losing weight and looking good, so don't dismiss this if your primary goal is a tight tush. What I'm asking you to do is take 30 days and eat more fruits and veggies instead of the grains. See how you do. Not so hard, right? And just to head you off at the pass, let's tackle two other grain related topics: "Whole grains" and Quinoa.

Whole grains are held up as some kind of miracle food, but did you guys read the Hunter Gatherers Are Us chapter? Have you been reading this grain chapter? Grains are NOT healthy! Be they whole or half a grain. You will see in a later chapter that grains are, calorie per calorie, remarkably weak as compared to lean meats, seafood, veggies, and fruit. You can look that stuff up yourself on the USDA nutrient database website. It's an eye-opener, especially for vegetarians. Now this is just considering the value of grains with regards to vitamins, minerals, and macronutrients like protein, carbs, and fat. When we factor in their anti-nutrient properties, and potential to wreck havoc on our GI tract, grains are not a sound decision for health or longevity.

Quinoa pops up frequently and the refrain goes like this, "Robb! Have you tried this stuff Quinoa (the pronunciation varies depending on how big a hippy you are). It's NOT a grain! It's fine, right?"

Well, you've likely heard the expression, "If it looks like a duck and quacks like a duck…" Quinoa is botanically not a grain, but because it has evolved in a similar biological niche, Quinoa has similar properties to grains, including chemical defense systems that irritate the gut. In the case of Quinoa, it contains soap-like molecules called saponins. Unlike gluten, which attaches to a carrier molecule in the intestines, saponins simply punch holes in the membranes of the microvilli cells. Yes, that's bad. Saponins are so irritating to the immune system that they are used in vaccine research to help the body mount a powerful immune response. The bottom line is if you think grains or grain-like items like Quinoa are healthy or benign, you are not considering the full picture. Follow the 30 day meal plan and see how you look, feel, and perform. Then you can speak from a place of experience.

One for Me and One for You

Some plants, like blueberries or similar fruits, have evolved a strategy of "give a little to get a little." Critters (us included) eat these fruits, then pass the seeds in a convenient, warm fertilized package that all but guarantees the next generation. Sewage systems aside, this is a reasonable trade off. The critter that eats the blueberries gets a little nutrition in exchange for spreading the blueberry seeds for subsequent generations of blueberries.

Other plants take a different approach and try to dissuade *all* predation by shrouding themselves in nasty substances that are either irritants or outright poisons. Consider poison oak or poison ivy. These plants have developed chemical warfare capabilities and use oils that have a tendency to work their way through the skin of animals that come in contact with the leaves. This oil sets off an alarm that irritates the immune system. Lymphocytes and other white blood cells attack the oil and in the process release pro-inflammatory chemicals that lead to a rash. Keep this idea in mind as we talk about grains, as it will help you to wrap your mind around what is happening when we eat this "staple" food.

If we compare grains to the strategies listed above, "give a little, get a little," like the blueberry, or "bugger off," like the poison oak, we see that grains are much more like poison oak. If a critter eats a grain, that's it for the grain. That does not mean that the grain goes down without a fight! Grains are remarkably well equipped for chemical warfare.

Lectins

Grains contain a variety of proteins, some of which are called lectins (not to be confused with the hormone leptin. Sorry folks, you need to stay on your toes!). In simple terms, lectins stick to specific molecules and thus play "recognition" roles in biological systems.

For our purposes, we will look at wheat germ agglutinin (WGA), which is one of the nastier lectins, but also one of the better studied. Keep in mind, WGA (or similar molecules) are found in *all* grains, but it's my opinion (and that of many other researchers) that wheat, rye, barley, and millet, which are the gluten-containing grains, are likely the worst of the bunch with regard to health. Corn and rice can be problematic, but they are safer if consumed infrequently (we will look at this later). WGA and similar lectins are problematic for several reasons:

1. Lectins are not broken down in the normal digestive process. This leaves large, intact proteins in the gut. If you recall, most proteins are broken down in the digestive process, but the structure of some grain proteins makes them very difficult to digest (for the geeks: these proteins are high in the amino acid proline). Grains also contain protease inhibitors (dairy and some other foods also contain these), which further block the digestion of dangerous lectins. This lack of adequate protein digestion leads to serious problems, as you will see.

2. The lectins attach to receptors in the intestinal lumen and are transported *intact* through the intestinal lining. Remember how amino acids and sugars are transported out of the intestines during digestion? Certain lectins "fool" transport molecules in an effort to gain entry into our bodies *intact.*

3. These large, intact protein molecules are easily mistaken by the body as foreign invaders like bacteria, viruses, or parasites. It's perhaps unpleasant to think about, but the intestines are not the nicest place to hang out. This area is a major source of infection by bacteria and viruses, and the immune system lies primed, waiting to pounce on any invading pathogen. Not only does WGA enter the system intact, it damages the intestinal lining, allowing other proteins to enter the system. Why is this a problem? Our immune system mounts an attack on these foreign proteins and makes antibodies against them. These antibodies are very specific to the shapes of these foreign proteins. Unfortunately, these proteins *also* tend to look like proteins in our body.

Brother from a Different Mother—Molecular Mimicry

As you recall, proteins are made of molecules called amino acids (AA). Let's imagine for a minute these amino acids are represented by Legos, with different shapes and colors denoting different amino acids. Imagine a string of Legos with a specific sequence; let's say its five to ten

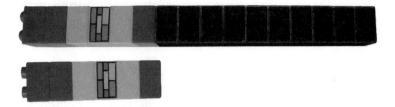

Legos long. Now imagine another, identical set of Legos attached on top of many more Legos. The top five to ten of the long piece is identical to the short piece. Let's assume the short piece is WGA and the long piece is a protein in the beta cells of your pancreas where insulin is made. If the WGA is attacked by the immune system and an antibody is made against it (because the body thinks WGA is a bacteria or virus), that antibody will not only attach to WGA, it can also attach to the protein in your pancreas. When that WGA antibody attaches to your pancreas, it precipitates a wholesale immune response—attacking that tissue. Your pancreas is damaged, or destroyed, and you become type 1 diabetic. If that protein happened to be in the myelin sheath of your brain, you would develop multiple sclerosis.

Celiac

Most people are familiar with a condition called celiac, which is an autoimmune disease caused by gluten, a protein found in wheat, rye, barley, and millet. It is clearly understood that celiac is an autoimmune disease caused by lectins. It is also clear that other autoimmune diseases such as rheumatoid arthritis, lupus, Sjögren's, multiple sclerosis, and a host of other autoimmune conditions occur at much higher rates in celiac patients. However, this association, for whatever reason, was largely dismissed as an anomaly until researchers recently made the connection between the development of celiac and other autoimmune diseases.

We now understood that WGA and other lectins have a significant effect on the enzyme transglutaminase (TG). Transglutaminase is an enzyme that modifies *every* protein we make in our body. How many proteins does TG modify folks? That's right, *all* of them. Heart, brain, kidney, reproductive organs—all of them. So, if lectins can cause problems with TG, and if TG modifies every protein in our body, how many things can lectins cause problems with? I hope this is obvious—lectins can and do affect every organ system. Reproductive issues, vitiligo (a skin condition where the individual loses pigmentation in the skin) Huntington's, narcolepsy—we have found literally hundreds of conditions in which lectins appear to be the causative factor. Not only do we have science to support this, we have observed clinical resolution of these conditions upon the removal of grains, legumes, and dairy. I hate to do this to you, but we have to go back into the intestines.

Really? Digestion? Again?

Yes, sorry about this, but we need to crawl back through the digestive tract. Don't worry; we will jump right in at the good stuff: the small intestines.

If you recall, when food is emptied from the stomach into the small intestines it is mixed with bile salts that are produced in the liver and stored in the gall bladder. Remember, bile salts are much like soap and are critical for our digestion and absorption of fats. In addition to bile from the gall bladder, the pancreas releases digestive enzymes that are critical to digestion. And lest you forget, much of the digestive process happens at the tiny structures in our intestines—the villi and microvilli. Now let's see how lectins interact with the intestinal lining to produce autoimmunity.

Lectins such as WGA bind to a receptor in the microvilli, allowing WGA to be transported into the body. This is the mechanism of the autoimmune cascade I described above. If the gut wall (microvilli) becomes damaged, the entire contents of the intestines can now make its way into your system. Yes, that's as bad as it sounds. You are not only in a position to create antibodies against WGA, which leads to autoimmunity, but you now have the potential to develop multiple allergies due to a permeable gut lining and inadequately digested food. This is how you can develop allergies to chicken, beef, apples, or other normally benign foods.

Additionally, if your gut is damaged, you expose yourself to a host of chemicals that would normally remain in the intestines. This can lead to conditions such as multiple chemical sensitivity syndrome, which is regarded more as a psychiatric problem than legitimate medical condition.

Let me be crystal clear about this: Anything that damages the gut lining (including bacterial, viral, and parasitic infections, as well as alcohol, grains, legumes, and dairy) can predispose one to autoimmunity, multiple chemical sensitivities, and allergies to otherwise benign foods.

As my Brazilian Jiu-Jitsu coach says, "This no opinion is, this fact is."
     "If the gut wall (microvilli) becomes damaged, the entire contents of the intestines can now make its way into your system."

Full of Bile

While this digestive disaster is taking place, there are several other problems brewing. As you recall, the function of the gall bladder is to release bile salts into a meal as it is emptied into the duodenum from the stomach. When the intestinal wall is damaged, the chemical messenger, cholecystokinin (CCK), is not released. CCK usually sends the "on" switch to the gall bladder and the secretion of pancreatic digestive enzymes. When this signal is blocked, we do not properly digest our foods, particularly fat and protein. The lack of bile release allows cholesterol crystals to form in the gall bladder, which leads to gall stones. The standard medical practice of removing the gall bladder is effectively killing the "canary in the coal mine." Gall stones are a symptom of a problem, an alarm. Instead of treating the cause (remove grains) we cut out the gall bladder. People who have had gall bladder removal are almost certainly undiagnosed celiacs and likely have a number of other progressive diseases. In my experience, these individuals are plagued with digestive problems, culminating in dysphagia, or difficulty swallowing.

Achtung!
The disruption of CCK and related hormones (PYY, adiponectin) in the signaling cascade of digestion is a really big deal. Not only is the digestive process severely damaged, much of our satiety signaling is

taken offline as well. We cannot properly digest our food, we are always "hungry," and the very food we crave, refined grains and sugary junk, happens to be the cause of the problem.

It Gets Better

Another piece of the chemical defense system used against us by grains is a group of enzymes called protease inhibitors. Protease inhibitors prevent the breakdown of proteins. This means that when you consume grains you do not effectively digest the protein in your meal. Protease inhibitors also stymie the digestion of lectins such as WGA, making these already difficult-to-digest items virtually indestructible. This leaves more large proteins in the intestinal contents, which increases our likelihood of developing autoimmunity, allergies, or chemical sensitivities.

Osteoporotic Much?

If you do not have a bellyache thinking about grains by now, let's look at one more player: antinutrients such as phytates. Phytates are important for seeds and grains because they tightly bind to metal ions (like magnesium, zinc, iron, calcium, and copper), which are crucial for the growth and development of the grain. If the metal ions are not tightly bound by the phytates, the process of germination can happen prematurely and this can spell disaster for the grain. When we consume grains, the phytates are still active and powerfully bind to calcium, magnesium, zinc, and iron. This means the calcium, magnesium, zinc, and iron are unavailable for absorption. Because of the action of antinutrients such as phytates combined with the gut damaging characteristics of lectins and protease inhibitors, our Neolithic ancestors lost an average of six inches in height vs. our Paleolithic ancestors due to the Neolithic diet of grains and legumes (remember the agriculturalists in chapter 2?). Are you concerned about osteoporosis or iron deficiency anemia? Do you suffer from fatigue or heart problems that might be caused by magnesium deficiency? Have you diligently consumed a "smart" diet of whole grains, legumes, and low-fat dairy as per the recommendations of your dietician and doctor? Do you see how ridiculous that suggestion is in light of what you now know about grains, legumes, and dairy?

Thank You Sir, May I Have Another!

Here is a recap of how grains cause malabsorption issues and how that affects our health and well-being:

1. Damage to the gut lining. If the gut is damaged, you do not absorb nutrients. We need healthy villi and microvilli to absorb our nutrients, be they protein, carbohydrates, fats, vitamins, or minerals.

2. Damage to the gall bladder and bile production. If you do not absorb fats and fat soluble nutrients such as vitamins A, D, K, and other nutrients, you will have problems utilizing any minerals you *do* absorb, to say nothing of the nutrient deficiencies from inadequate essential fats.

3. Phytates tightly bind to metal ions and make them unavailable for absorption. Analytical chemists actually use purified phytates in experiments where it is necessary to quantify the amounts of metal ions like calcium, zinc, or iron in a sample because the phytates bind to these metals tighter than just about any other molecule. The same thing happens when you eat phytates, and this is *not* a good thing for bone health or iron status.

4. Open door for autoimmunity and cancer. Once the gut lining is damaged, we are at exceptionally high risk of autoimmune disease, such as Hashimoto's thyroiditis, and several types of cancer, including non-Hodgkin's lymphoma. The pancreas is assailed by grain-induced inflammation due to CCK problems and elevated insulin levels. This inflammation is a potential cause of pancreatic cancer and pancreatitis (inflammation of the pancreas).

Why does all this happen? Because grains are pissed that you want to eat them and they are willing, and able, to fight back.

Here is a *short* list of the problems associated with leaky gut and the autoimmune response:
- Infertility
- Type 1 diabetes

- Multiple sclerosis
- Rheumatoid Arthritis
- Lupus
- Vitiligo
- Narcolepsy
- Schizophrenia
- Autism
- Depression
- Huntington's
- Non-Hodgkin's lymphoma
- Hypothyroidism
- Porphyria

Yeah, But I'm Not Sick

Like I said, this is a short list of the issues we know are tied to autoimmunity and that have shown improvement or complete resolution when one eats in accordance with the recommendations in this book. When we get to the prescriptive chapter, I'll provide detailed guidelines to help give you the best chance at reversing or preventing these and other problems.

Some of you, however, may think you have no issues here. You have eaten grains, legumes, and dairy your whole life and are "fine." Well, maybe. But I suspect that is not the case. I'll bet that if you completely remove these Neolithic foods from your diet for one month, you will notice a dramatic improvement in how you feel and perform. Why? Because if you are consuming these foods, I'll wager you have gut irritation and other systemic inflammation issues.

A recent study looking at children with type 1 diabetes (an autoimmune condition) found that a significant number of them had overt gut pathology, i.e., celiac. Some had a positive antibody test for celiac, but a number of kids were negative on both the WGA antibody test (a common blood test for celiac) and on an intestinal biopsy. So doctors would think there was no gluten influence in their condition. Interestingly, however, nearly all the kids showed antibodies in the deep tissues of the microvilli to . . . transglutaminase.

The study authors suspected most of the kids would at some point develop what is commonly described as celiac. What this tells us is gut damage can be fairly benign (few symptoms) but still lead to autoimmunity. Once initiated, autoimmunity can and does progress to other problems. Your doctor or dietician will likely dismiss this information, especially if you are "negative" for any of the standard blood work or lab tests for celiac. They are foolish in this regard, but hey, it's only *your* health.

Trust your medical professionals, they always know best. Or, try a simple experiment: Follow a Paleo diet, and assess how you feel and perform. I know, I can hear the MDs now, that it's "just anecdotal." If you are going to save your ass you are not likely to get much support in this matter unless you have a forward-thinking and aggressive primary physician.

What is the ultimate gold standard in all this? How do you know for sure you do or do not have an issue with these foods? The answer seems obvious: remove the potentially offending foods! Reintroduce them after thirty to sixty days. See what happens. Now there is a caveat to this. You only need to be exposed to things like gluten once every ten to fifteen days to keep the gut damaged. This can bedevil people as they "cut back on gluten" but do not notice an improvement in their overall health. I'm sorry but there is not a pink "participant" ribbon given out for doing this "almost correctly." You need to be 100 percent compliant for thirty days, then see how you do with reintroduction.

Now, I'll be honest, the reintroduction is for *you*, not me. If I did a phone consult with you, I'd ask, "How did you do when you had that piece of bread?" I know exactly how you did—I've seen this scenario thousands of times, but *you* are the one who needs convincing. When you reintroduce gluten you will not feel good. Sorry kiddo, it's just the way it works. Now it's up to you to decide if health and a long life are worth forgoing some of these foods more often than not.

Does all this seem hard to believe? Well, remember how I described the effects of poison oak on your skin? It's a similar deal here with gut irritation and lectin exposure. If you want to get the full power of this program, you need to actually give it a shot. Worst-case scenario: You spend a month without some foods you like. Best-case scenario: You discover you are able to live healthier and better than you ever thought possible. If you cannot suck it up for a month to discover that, well, Buttercup, you might be beyond help. And let's be honest, most of your arguments have *nothing* to do with the science—you are likely addicted to these foods.

But I Like Bread and Pasta!

Yes, I like that stuff too, but they make me sick. I suspect it makes you sick, as well. Not only do grains make you sick by raising insulin levels, messing up your fatty acid ratios (n-3/n-6), and irritating your gut, but they are also addictive. Grains, particularly the gluten-containing grains, contain molecules that fit into the opiate receptors in our brain. You know, the same receptors that work with heroine, morphine, and Vicodin? Most people can take or leave stuff like corn tortillas and rice. Suggest that people should perhaps forgo bread and pasta for their health and they will bury a butter knife in your forehead before you can say "whole wheat!" Sorry folks, I don't make these rules, I just have the lovely task of educating you about them.

Why I had to focus on gluten-free living, exercise, and trying to get you healthy, I will never know. I should have just peddled hookers, cocaine, and pastries! So much easier.

But, But, But!

Egad! I can hear it now: What about *whole grains?* What about *brown* rice? What about Ezekial Bread? What about the China Study? What about fiber and vitamins? Want more science, more convincing? To this I have one word: *Do.*

I could make this book a thousand pages of science and technical investigation, but someone could still find a stone I have left unturned. This is a stalling technique, nothing more. If you want to be healthier, look better, and perform better, you need to *do*. Ultimately, it is your personal experience that matters. Want more science? Want to argue about it? Read *every* citation I have in this book, the published research on my website, and then come to town, buy me a NorCal margarita, and be ready for a chat. But first, you still need to go thirty days grain, legume, and dairy free. I have "tried it" your way. Take thirty days, do it my way, then tell me what happened. Read the literature and be articulate in the science, and have thirty days of personal experience to speak from. Arm-chair quarterbacks do not get a say in the matter, capisce?

Listen, I'm not trying to be a jerk here. I'm trying to help improve, possibly save, *your* life. This book is full of "science," but none of that matters compared to your personal experience. Get in, do it, and then evaluate critically, OK?

I will lay out how to do this. I will show the nutrient inferiority of grains compared to fruits and vegetables (I hear fruits and veggies have vitamins, minerals, and even this wacky stuff called fiber. Apparently, this info has not been passed along to registered dieticians). I will show what to expect with regard to fat loss and what lab values to track. It's easy to do. It may be new to you, but you can do it. Put down that cookie! It's time to learn about fat.

Legumes and Dairy

Believe it or not, I don't want to bury you with technical details, but I'm trying to tell you what you *need* in order to understand the material. With this in mind, it is important to address the topics of legumes (lentils, beans . . . you know, fun foods that make you toot!) and dairy.

In simple terms, dairy and legumes have problems similar to grains: Gut irritating proteins, antinutrients, and protease inhibitors. In rheumatology circles, it has long been understood that bean sprouts are highly problematic for folks with autoimmune diseases such as rheumatoid arthritis and lupus. Some doctors have made the connection to dairy as well. I could have included a chapter similar to the one I did on grains for both dairy and legumes, but to what effect other than burying you with repetitious material? In an effort to prevent brain implosion from information overload, you need to understand that these foods are also on the thirty-day "no fly" list.

I've included research in the reference section specific to the autoimmune and metabolic problems associated with dairy and legumes. So, if you want to geek-out on that stuff, by all means go for it. What you will find are mechanisms eerily similar to grains: Gut irritation, protease inhibitors, antinutrients, and inflammation. When we get to the prescriptive chapter, I will walk you through specifically what items to avoid, and how you can tinker with the occasional reintroduction of these foods.

PS. OK, I have this sneaky suspicion you're going to be slippery about this topic. As you will see in the prescriptive chapter, it is critical that you consider grains, legumes, and dairy all in the same category. This is particularly true if you have weight loss goals, inflammation, or autoimmunity. Yes, honey, cut the cheese.

SEVEN

◇◇

Fat
Have a Seat, This May Take a Little While

◇◇

One night I took my wife Nicki out to our favorite Thai restaurant. You would likely walk right by the place fearing some significant health code violations, but this little hole-in-the-wall is amazing and typical of the best eateries: All the love is in the food, not fancy décor. Our waiter was a college student we had seen several times on previous curry-binges, but this was the first time he waited on our table. He is a very upbeat kid, boisterous, funny, and pretty damn overweight. He seated us, made some small talk, and then asked us for our order:

• 2 orders of chicken satay (chicken skewers that are marinated in coconut milk and spices.
• 2 fresh coconuts (these are young coconuts full of water and with a jelly-like consistency on the inside. AMAZING).
• 2 orders of red curry. Mine mild, Nicki's medium-hot.
• Instead of rice, we asked for a steamed vegetable medley that included carrots, broccoli, several types of mushrooms, and bamboo shoots. Part of why we love this place is they give us over a pound of steamed veggies instead of rice.

Our very nice, very funny, very overweight waiter looked perplexed, almost upset. I thought it was because Nicki and I have the annoying couples' habit of ordering the same things. No, our waiter was concerned for our health. Our overweight waiter said to Nicki and me, "Are you guys *trying* to stop your hearts?"

I still left him a tip, just not a large one.

Nicki and I are in pretty damn good shape and our blood work leaves our doctors jabbering about how we will "live forever." All is well until the discussion of what we actually eat. Then we get the same look from the doctor as from our waiter. Our waiter was convinced that our high-fat meal, particularly of high saturated fat from coconut, was going to kill us before we finished eating. Our doctor was (and is) convinced we were ticking time bombs, just waiting for the day when our blood chemistries take a turn for the dead.

Oy-vey!

Fat Confusion

This chapter has proven to be one of the toughest for me to write because I was stumped where the hell to start. People seem to generally understand the insulin/refined carbs concept. Kinda. People have heard of low-carb, perhaps even dabbled with it, but even though most of you are OK with the idea that refined carbs are bad, you still think fat is bad. Our governmental agencies have done a great job of convincing us that fat, particularly animal fat, is pure evil. We were told to cut fat, increase "complex carbs," and all would be well. That is true if you are in the business of coronary artery bypass, statins, diabetes meds, or gastric bypass.

The government high-carb, low-fat fantasy is turning out to be amazingly profitable for sectors of our medical and pharmaceutical establishment. Unfortunately, it's not been kind to our friends, family, and coworkers.

I'm going to touch on the history of this story because it's a reasonable question to ask, "How did seemingly smart people make such a dumb mistake?" I will not, however, do an exhaustive analysis of this multibillion-dollar farce. If you want a full accounting, check out the books *Protein Power* and *Good Calories, Bad Calories*. It seems silly for me to rehash the details of this medical history, as I would prefer to focus on how to *fix* your situation. So, if you want to dig deeper on this topic, check out the aforementioned books and the resources in the appendix. For now we will look at how the McGovern Commission has cost us billions of dollars and millions of lives.

Remember, the reason why we need to look at all this is because you, your doctor, and your uncle Fred will ask the probing question, "Won't eating fat kill you?" I wish I could just put people in a headlock and give them a noogie until they agreed to try the recommendations in the book, but my parole officer and lawyer have explained to me this constitutes "assault." Hence, the science.

Ancel Keys and the McGovern Commission

In the early 1950s a biochemist named Ancel Keys submitted a paper for publication titled, "The Seven Countries Study." This was an early bit of epidemiological work that appeared to show a strong statistical relationship between the amount of fat consumed in a given country and the incidence of heart attack. It *appeared* to be an airtight case that the more fat a country consumed, the more heart disease. In fact, the data Keys reported did follow this trend line, but only when he conveniently *threw out* all of the conflicting results!

Numerous countries with high fat intake also showed remarkably low CVD. Other countries showed high CVD while eating little fat. When considered in its entirety, the Seven Countries Study should have involved twenty-two countries, and the conclusion from this larger (accurate) data set would have been, "There is no relationship between fat intake and CVD. Some other factor must be at play here."

Unfortunately, this is not what happened. Keys had a bit of a puritanical streak and felt people needed to restrict their rich food intake, particularly meat and saturated fat.

Keys recommended a "prudent diet" based on vegetable oils (like corn and soy) and grains, thus *theoretically* emulating the diet seen in the Mediterranean countries of Italy and Greece, both of which sported better average health than North America. Unfortunately, neither Keys nor anyone else noticed that the recommended "Mediterranean" diet looked nothing like the diets the French, Italians, and Greeks actually *ate*.

You Can't Eat a Meme

Good and bad ideas alike gain footholds largely because they are, to use Malcolm Gladwell's term, "sticky." People are exposed to the ideas, like them, and for good or ill, pass them along. Take this sticky idea, add capricious gods or dumb luck, and we have set the stage for toppling governments or killing millions of people because of bad policy.

In this situation, the idea that fat was the cause of CVD (eventually fat would be both condemned and subsequently acquitted of being the cause for cancer, cognitive decline, and host of other ills) was appealing to people. In addition to this, we had a post–World War II sense of government do-goodery that drove the McGovern Commission to champion the fat-heart hypothesis. This occurred despite massive outcry from the scientific community that dietary fat, in particular saturated fat, was *not* the causative factor in CVD. In a congressional hearing, scientists voiced their concerns over these sweeping, low-fat recommendations. In return, McGovern quipped that senators do not have the luxury of scientists, who wait for all the data to come "in" before making a decision. *Something* needed to be done!

So, we had one part "cooked" scientific data (which scored Keys a *Time* magazine cover), and one part governmental do-goodery. This might not have been enough to breathe this lipid-heart hypothesis monster into life, but we had one other unfortunate problem: human gullibility. Researchers reasoned that if Americans were fat, and suffering from more heart disease than other countries, they should reduce the fat in the diet. It was like a balanced chemical equation:

Fat in the diet = FAT People

Or, for the visual learners:

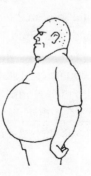

In support of this fat = fat idea, people like to throw around big words like "thermodynamics." Fat has more calories (9 calories/gram) than protein and carbohydrate (4 calories/gram). If one consumes more calories than one burns, this will lead to weight gain. So, reduce fat, and the likelihood of consuming too many calories would be reduced. This idea makes sense. It made so much sense that no one bothered to actually do their homework and make sure it was actually *true*. No one considered that carbohydrate, and the insulin it releases, drives hunger and fat storage. Also overlooked was the fact that protein and fat reduced total calorie intake by increasing satiety via PYY, adiponectin, and similar appetite-control mechanisms.

As I mentioned previously, researchers quickly discovered a number of "paradoxes" among people like the French, Spanish, and Greeks, who ate significantly more fat than Americans, yet were slimmer and suffered a fraction the CVD. We were so blinded by our fat phobia we could not see the facts for what they were. Instead we have tried to hang the health of the French and Greeks on things like red wine and olive oil.

If You Meet the Paradox on the Road . . .

There are no paradoxes in biology, only our mistaken assumptions about biology. The assumption that fat makes people fat and causes heart disease makes sense, but that does not make it *true*. In every clinical trial performed, carbohydrate-controlled (low-carb) diets provide more weight loss and better cardiovascular disease prevention than high-carb, low-fat alternatives. High-carb pundits keep peddling this failed approach, but it's as simple as trying the various approaches for one month so you can see which one allows you to look, feel, and perform your best.

The story above is a brief history of the inaccuracies surrounding the lipid-hypothesis and, honestly, it just scratches the surface. We have over fifty years of failed governmental policy to keep track of and millions of lives lost in the process. If you want to dig deeper on this topic, the resources mentioned above, along with those in the appendix, are waiting for you. Now, however, we need to look at what fat actually *does* do with regard to our performance, health, and longevity.

Fats! Bomp, Bomp, Bomp! What Are They Good For?

For most of us, fat is a dirty word. It's something that makes our fanny look terrible in a bikini. A few enlightened folks recognize that fat is important as a fuel and is a building block for many of our cell membranes and hormones. However, the reality is that fat is far more than just fuel or raw materials. It is us. Our brains are mainly fat, most of our nerves are fat. Reproductive hormones, yep, fat. Now there are different types of fat, and we will look at those sub-types because, if you can believe it, there are even *essential fats*. Fats that if you do not get enough of, or the right ratios, you will become sick or die.

When considering fats, it's helpful to understand just a little bit about their chemical structures. This is because their names and their physiological actions are tied to their structures. Fats come in varying lengths and they are divided into one of three general categories: saturated, monounsaturated, and polyunsaturated.

Now, most of you have heard the terms saturated and monounsaturated. Some of you might have even heard of polyunsaturated fats. What the names indicate is how many, if any, double bonds exist in a given fat. This is important because double bonds (or saturation), along with chain-length, are what separate one fat from another.

Stearic acid, for example, is an 18-carbon fat that contains no double bonds. In chemist geek speak, it is "saturated" with hydrogen, hence the name. In the case of oleic acid, we have an 18-carbon molecule with one double bond, which earns oleic acid the term *monounsaturated*. Finally, we have a fat like alpha-linolenic acid, which is also an 18-carbon-long molecule, but in this case it has several double bonds. We have arrived at the "polyunsaturated" fats.

As a final wrinkle, fats are usually bonded three at a time to an alcohol-like molecule called glycerol. This folks is what we call a triglyceride. If we eat something like steak, olive oil, or coconut, we take in triglycerides that are made up of different fatty acids. Most foods have a characteristic mix of fats, but some variation does occur, as we will see with the difference between grass-fed and grain-fed meats.

The chemical and physical properties of fats (are they liquid or solid at room temperature, do they go rancid (oxidize) easily or not?)

are dramatically altered by how long the molecule is *and* by how many (if any) double bonds are present in a particular fat. Saturated fats tend to be inert. Coconut oil, which is mainly a short-chain saturated fat, does not go bad even when exposed to the air for years. Linseed oil, by contrast, is a polyunsaturated fat that oxidizes so quickly one can start a fire by leaving linseed oil on things like rags or paper. Monounsaturated fats, not surprisingly, fall between the other two fats in how rapidly they go bad. I *know* you were dying to learn all this stuff. You will be ready to impress friends, family, and colleagues with your newfound knowledge. Feel smug.

Keep in mind that if you just want to reap the benefits of a Paleo diet, you need not understand any of the science and technical stuff. The reason I need to go into this level of detail, however, is because many people are confused about topics like saturated fat, cholesterol, and heart disease. Most of our lay populace, and seemingly even more of our medical community, are out to lunch on this topic. This forces me to get fairly detailed so you have an opportunity to understand all this. If I do a good job, it should allow you to read this book, implement the recommendations, track your progress, and, *ideally*, have few questions because I did my job up front. That's the idea, anyway. We'll see how effective I am. I mention this because we have a little more technical material to carve through before you will get your fifth-level "lipid-Jedi" decoder ring and start saving the world from the forces of evil: VEGANS!

What Fats Do What?

Different fats have different physiological roles. To keep things simple, I will only cover the fats most commonly occurring in the diet. Let's look at these fats from the perspective of the fat's level of saturation just to keep things tidy. This is also helpful as our first family of fats is more misunderstood than an Emo kid growing up in Arkansas.

Saturated Fats and Their Functions

Saturated fats have generated a bad rap over the years. Initially, they were saddled with the dubious distinction of being the cause of CVD. Then, researchers tried in vain to attach them to everything ranging from cancer to neurodegeneration. The reality is saturated fats are generally pretty benign, some actually helpful. All of them have been quite misunderstood. Let's look at the saturated fats starting with the short varieties, and then working our way longer.

Lauric Acid

Lauric acid is a 12-carbon-long saturated fat commonly found in coconut, palm oil, and, interestingly, human breast milk. Lauric acid has novel antiviral properties that include proven activity against HIV, chicken pox, cytomegalovirus, and many other viruses. Lauric acid also has properties that help to heal gut irritation, which we will see, is an important feature in reversing leaky gut and autoimmune issues. Lauric acid *can* increase LDL and thus, total cholesterol, but as you have learned, LDL cholesterol is relatively benign if we have low systemic inflammation and low insulin levels via limited carbohydrate intake.

Many populations, such as the extensively studied Kitavans, consume large amounts of Lauric acid, display higher cholesterol levels than other populations, yet suffer little CVD. Yet again it would appear nature has dealt us a paradox, but it was only our assumption that all saturated fat is bad that led us to this false conclusion.

Palmitic Acid

Palmitic acid is 16 carbons long, fully saturated, and commonly found in palm oil and animal products, including beef, eggs, milk, poultry, and seafood. Palmitic acid has long been implicated in CVD, as it tends to raise LDL cholesterol. Among the saturated fats, it would appear palmitic acid does pose the greatest likelihood of increasing LDL cholesterol. However, palmitic acid has also recently been shown to be vital both to forming new memories and accessing long-held memories. As we shall see when we investigate how our diet has changed, a Paleo diet supplies an adequate amount of palmitic acid for optimum cognitive function while limiting the intake to levels that are not harmful to the cardiovascular system. It is also important to note that excessive carbohydrate intake leads to palmitic acid production. If you recall from the insulin chapter, when liver glycogen is full, additional carbohydrate is converted to palmitic acid. This process appears to blunt our sensitivity to leptin, which then inhibits our satiety to a normal meal.

This is the beginning of insulin resistance and is at the heart of the mechanism of how we cease to respond to food by feeling "full."

Stearic Acid

The final saturated fat we will consider is the 18-carbon stearic acid. Stearic acid is found in significant amounts in meat, eggs, and chocolate! Stearic acid appears to be neutral with regard to LDL number, but it has been shown to actually increase HDL levels. Stearic acid also decreases a marker of systemic inflammation, Apollo protein-A.

Saturated Fat: The Bottom Line, Please

Even though this was a quick sprint through the saturated fats, it was likely still enough to send some folks into a fetal position. So, what *is* the bottom line here? Are saturated fats bad or not? Do they increase the potential for CVD? Well, it depends.

A high intake of saturated fats, in conjunction with a high intake of dietary carbohydrate, is a hell of a combo for an early grave. As you saw in previous chapters, elevated insulin levels lead to a shift in the LDL particles to a type that is small, dense, and easily oxidized. This is bad for a number of reasons, but the central feature is increased systemic inflammation and a subsequent increased probability of a cardiovascular event like heart attack or stroke. *No bueno.* If, however, our intake of saturated fat is kept within ancestral limits, *and* we also modify our carbohydrate intake to match that of our ancestors (both in amounts and type), we have little if any risk of developing CVD. We will look at the specifics of this after we have tackled mono and poly-unsaturated fats.

Monounsaturated Fats

Really, this section should be titled "monounsaturated fat" because although there are a number of monos (the acronym is MUFA—monounsaturated fatty acid), we are really concerned with only one variety, called oleic acid. Oleic is an 18-carbon-long MUFA found mainly in plant sources, such as olive oil, avocados, and nuts. Don't count animal sources out, however! Even grain-fed meat contains a significant amount of oleic. Most people are familiar with the Mediterranean diet, and much of the health benefits ascribed to the diet are centered on the "heart healthy" MUFAs. Indeed, MUFAs are pretty impressive with regards to their benefits: Improved insulin sensitivity, improved glucagon response, and decreased cholesterol levels. Most plant sources of MUFA are also accompanied by fat-soluble antioxidants that are incorporated into the membranes of our cells, thus preventing oxidative damage associated with aging and most degenerative diseases. MUFAs were the primary fat in our ancestral diet, so if we want to optimize our performance, health, and longevity (and look good naked), we will construct meals that emphasize this cornerstone of the Paleo diet.

Polyunsaturated Fats: AKA the Essential Fats

As paradoxical as it may sound, there are indeed essential fats. We cannot make them and must consequently get them from our diet. If you do not get enough of these fats *or* the right ratios, you will have *big* problems. For our international readers, that's *Problemas Grandes,* or *Scheissen Grossen!* As you will see, they are not only essential, but they also represent one of the largest divergences from our ancestral diet and into our corn-fed catastrophe. The next section will look at two subfamilies of polyunsaturated fats (PUFA) called the omega-3 family and the omega-6 family (abbreviated as n-3 and n-6 respectively). Sit tight folks, if you have not fallen asleep yet, you will soon!

Key Points

Just to keep you on track, here are the key points that you should take away from the forthcoming section. These bullet points will help you make sense of the science-laden geek-speak that will be poured on you like a scalding beaker full of grass-fed beef stew.

1. Long n-3/n-6s are good. We get these from grass-fed meats and wild-caught fish.
2. Ancestral ratios of n-3/n-6 were approximately 1 to 1. Modern ratios are 1 to 10. This is bad.
3. Corn, soy, safflower, and similar vegetable oils are the source of the excessive n-6 fats in our diet.

Give Me a 3!

Alpha-Linolenic Acid (ALA)

ALA is a short (18-carbon) n-3 found in flax, hemp, and other plant sources. It is sub-par for our goals of enhancing performance, health, and longevity. It is adequate to the needs of keeping vegetarian hippies alive (I guess that's a good thing), but we are much more interested in EPA and DHA, found only from animal sources, such as wild fish and game, certain types of eggs (from chickens fed flax seed), and grass-fed meat. If you look at the attached diagram, you will notice that ALA can be converted to EPA and DHA, but it is a painfully inefficient process. Like I said, ALA will keep you alive—it will not allow you to thrive.

Eicosapentaenoic Acid (EPA)

EPA is a 20-carbon-long PUFA that is vital to life. Like I mentioned previously, it *can* be manufactured from the shorter-chain ALA, but it is a slow process and there are downsides associated with ALA, which we will discuss in a moment. EPA is a potent anti-inflammatory, decreases platelet aggregation (thins the blood), and blocks angiogenesis (the growth of new blood vessels, one of the mechanisms necessary for cancer to spread). In non-geek speak *¡EPA es muy bueno!*

Docosahexaenoic Acid (DHA)

DHA is a 22-carbon PUFA that is critical for fetal brain development and normal cognitive functions throughout life. Mothers who have inadequate stores of DHA are at particularly high risk of deficiency during pregnancy and postpartum. For the child, this can mean stunted neurological development. For the mother, this can mean dramatically increased susceptibility to complications such as preeclampsia, gestational diabetes, and postpartum depression. Similar to EPA, DHA has potent antitumor and anti-inflammatory actions. Our bodies can interconvert EPA to DHA and vice versa, but we appear to run best when we have ample amounts of both essential fats.

OK, time to look at the omega-6 family of essential fats.

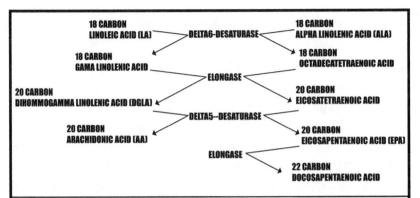

This is a paired-downed graphic representing conversion of short-chain n-3/n-6 fatty acids to longer chain n-3/n-6 fats. Our physiology is wired for a dynamic equilibreum built from n-3/n-6 ratios ranging from 1-1 to 1-2. The n-3/n-6 fats share the various enzymes listed above. An overabundance of one fatty acid family can dramatically impair the conversion of the alternate family. Our modern diet with its Omega 6 dominance impedes the production of the long-chain Omega 3 family and their anti-inflammatory by-products, including Prostaglandins. This is also why some otherwise favorable Paleo foods like nuts and seeds can be problematic, as they frequently have much greater Omega 6 content, which can push your dietary fatty acid ratios to a pro-inflammatory (n-6 heavy) state.

To avoid problems, mainly use nuts and seeds as you would a condiment.

"Red Leader . . . I've Got Your 6!"

Linoleic Acid

Linoleic acid (LA) is an 18-carbon n-6 PUFA found in high concentration in vegetable oils such as safflower and sunflower. Both LA and its longer metabolites are potent mediators of systemic inflammation (i.e., they are pro-inflammatory). As we will see, this makes some otherwise "Paleo" foods such as certain nuts problematic because LA can block the anti-inflammatory effects of EPA and DHA. This is also why corn, sunflower, and soy oils are so bad for us, as they are loaded with LA. Let's take a look at the metabolites of LA.

Gamma Linolenic Acid

Gamma linolenic acid (GLA) is an 18-carbon n-6 PUFA with one more double bond than LA. Dietary sources of GLA include borage, primrose, and hemp oils. The body can convert LA into GLA, but this process can decrease in the case of hyperinsulinism and viral infection. As you will see, the n-6 family of PUFAs tend to be pro-inflammatory. However, GLA can act as an anti-inflammatory agent (as compared to LA) by blocking the production of various prostaglandins. Hang in there, just a few more!

Dihomo-Gamma-Linolenic Acid

Dihomo gamma-linolenic acid (DGLA) is a 20-carbon n-6 PUFA. DGLA regulates the production of several important families of molecular messengers including series 1 thromboxanes and leukotrienes—molecules crucial in the regulation of immune function, inflammation, and pain. DGLA is produced from GLA and can be converted into arachidonic acid, the final n-6 PUFA we will consider.

Arachidonic Acid

Arachidonic acid (AA) is a 20-carbon n-6 PUFA found predominately in animal products. It regulates a host of metabolic functions via actions on prostaglandins, thromboxanes, and leukotrienes. AA gets a bad rap because it is involved in metabolic pathways largely controlling inflammation. This is a mistake. AA is critical for normal actions such as adapting to exercise, muscle repair, and brain function. Think of AA like daytime television: vital to life, but also toxic in excessive amounts.

OK, So What?

I know this is a ton of information, but like I said previously, I need to cover all of this material for one main reason:

I need to answer all the inaccuracies that form the basis of our governmental and academic nutritional recommendations. You are bombarded by government information pushing a grain-based, high-carb, low-fat diet. They are wrong and I need to detail *why* they are wrong; otherwise you are trading one false god for another.

In the prescriptive chapter, I will provide concrete guidelines for assessing just how well a Paleo diet works for restoring health and vigor. I will describe objective lab values that prove a Paleo diet is the best way you can fuel yourself. I wish we could just jump in and hit the "how to" material, but I need to answer questions about saturated fat, essential fats, and these myriad related topics so *you* can understand just how all this works.

When we consider fats and their potential impact on health and disease, our Paleo Solution can help us by providing guidelines that helps us make sense of dietary fat.

• **No trans fats.** Our ancestors never saw a trans fat.* The concept of trans fats is only about fifty years old and our metabolism has no idea what to do with them. Trans fats are created when polyunsaturated fats from corn, soybean, and similar oils are exposed to heat, hydrogen gas, and a catalyst. The resulting fat looks and acts similar to saturated fats (it does not go rancid quickly, so it is solid or semisolid at room temperature), but with some serious flaws: Trans fats ruin liver function. They wreak havoc on blood lipids. They destroy insulin sensitivity. Want to die young? Eat plenty of trans fats and high-fructose corn syrup (soda and chips anyone?) and your family can collect on your life insurance in short order.

Trans fats *should* become less of a problem over time, as they are being phased out of restaurants and prepared foods. The irony is trans fats were used as a replacement for supposedly harmful fats such as coconut and palm oil. The same governmental do-goodery that brought us the high-carb, low-fat diet, also brought us trans fats. Interestingly, both recommendations strongly support the subsidized agriculture scene in the United States. Although palm oil may be high in palmitic acid, and thus not the greatest option, it is far better than Franken-foods like hydrogenated vegetable oils and margarine.

So, trans fats should be: 0%. By the way, when the government comes to help you, run. They are either bringing a firing squad or dietary changes, but the end result is the same.

---

* You will notice that a nutritional breakdown of grass-fed meat shows a small amount of trans fats. Should you panic? Is there some kind of mistake? No, this is normal and, ironically, healthy. The trans fats produced in wild or grass-fed meat products is naturally occurring and actually healthy. They include fats such as conjugated linoleic acid (CLA), which has proven anticancer and antioxidant activities and improves muscle growth and leanness. The bottom line is that trans fats in grass-fed meat are *not* a problem.

- **Amount of Fat.** Total fat intake appears to have little bearing on most health and disease. We see populations with as low as 10 percent fat intake and as high as 50 percent fat intake with similar CVD rates. We will tinker with your intake to see what works best for you.

- **Types of fat.** Type of fat appears to bear strongly on disease processes, but the key players have changed. Saturated fat has historically been implicated as a causative factor in everything from CVD to cancer. However, closer analysis has shown this assumption to be largely inaccurate. When we consider our ancestral diet, we see saturated fats tended to account for 10–15 percent of total fat intake in most populations. Exceptions to this include populations near sources of coconut (lauric acid). In these populations, we may see intake of saturated fat as high as 40 percent of calories, but none of these hunter-gatherer populations show significant signs of CVD. One key feature of the hunter-gatherer diet is a low total palmitic acid content. So, although palmitic acid does appear to increase LDL cholesterol, other factors appear more important in CVD propagation. The n-3/n-6 fats appear to play the primary role in disease processes such as cancer, diabetes, autoimmunity, and neurodegeneration.

- **Saturated fat.** Our ancestral diet *did* have saturated fat, but as you will see, it was seldom a large percentage of calories. Additionally, the saturated fat in a Paleolithic diet tended to be cardio-neutral fats, such as stearic and lauric acids. Due to grain feeding of our meat, we consume far more palmitic acid, which can increase LDL cholesterol. Although this is not the only risk factor in CVD, it is something we can easily modify by emulating a Paleolithic diet using modern foods such as grass-fed meat and wild-caught fish.

- **Omega-3 vs. Omega-6 essential fatty acids.** N-3/n-6 fats are important in *every* aspect of inflammation. N-3/n-6 fats also control elements of cancer, Parkinson's, Alzheimer's, and fertility. Anything in which inflammation plays a role. And, that's actually about everything. If you recall from the description of essential fats, n-3s are broadly categorized as anti-inflammatory, whereas n-6's are generally pro-inflammatory (there are some exceptions to this, but it works for our purposes). The crux of the problem is this: Our ancestral diet provided about one omega-3 fat for every one or two omega-6 fats. Our genetics are therefore designed for about equal amounts of pro and anti-inflammatory signals from the fats in our diet. Our *current* diet has a ratio of about one omega-3 fat for every ten to twenty omega-6 fats. The signal to our body has been shifted massively toward the pro-inflammatory side of the equation and, not surprisingly, we are not doing so well with the change.

How do we get things right again? Focus on grass-fed and wild-caught fish, avoid sources of n-6 fats especially some seed and grain oils, and supplement with some fish oil. We will talk about how much fish oil to take a little later.

Fat Wrap

Hopefully you are getting a sense of why we are so concerned with n-3 and n-6 fatty acids. They are key players in controlling hormone-like substances with sexy names like prostaglandins, thromboxanes, leukotrienes, endocannabinoids, cytokines, and eicosanoids. These substances are the focus of billions of dollars per year in pharmaceutical sales and research because they control cell-to-cell communication throughout the body related to inflammation. Drugs that act on metabolic pathways such as the COX-1 and COX-2 (cyclooxygenase one and two respectively) include Viox, Celebrex, and our old friend aspirin. The COX pathways regulate much of what we perceive as pain and inflammation. It is impossible to overstate how powerful these substances are. They are all controlled by n-3/n-6 fats, insulin levels, and lifestyle issues, such as sleep and stress. What this means is we have significant control over these processes and can use our knowledge to forestall aging, cognitive decline, and a host of other degenerative disease.

Do You Need to Track What Types of Fats You Are Eating?

Not really. If you follow the simple meal plan we have in the book, you will be set. There is no need to micromanage this stuff if you follow the simple and delicious recipes and concepts of the Paleo Solution. As I've said before, you do not need to understand these concepts to *do* them, but you, your family, and your doctor will have questions, so you might as well have answers.

All that silly health stuff aside, if you balance your essential fats you will not only be healthy, you will lose fat, gain muscle (if you want to), have loads of energy, and generally feel good. Or in more compelling terms, your fanny will look great in a bikini. Or board shorts. However you roll!

Below is a list of n-3 super foods. If you want to really broaden your geek fat knowledge, check out Professor Cordain's website: http://www.thepaleodiet.com/nutritional_tools/fats.shtml

- Wild Alaskan Salmon
- Sardines
- Anchovies
- Mackerel
- Herring
- Trout
- Grass-Fed Meat
- Omega-3 Enriched Eggs

So Robb, this is the fat chapter, but you did not talk a lot about cholesterol. What's up?

Well, I did mention how palmitic acid can increase LDL count, but the reality is dietary carbohydrates have a much more important influence on cholesterol and overall cardiovascular disease risk. Here are a few things to remember with regard to excessive dietary carbohydrate and consequent hyperinsulinism:

- LDL cholesterol is converted to the small, dense atherogenic profile under the influence of excessive carbs.

• Total cholesterol is increased due to the up-regulation of HMG-COA reductase.

• Systemic inflammation is increased by up-regulation of pro-inflammatory prostaglandins, cytokines, and leukotrienes.

When considering cholesterol and CVD, the important points are:

• Focus on the amounts and types of dietary carbohydrates, emphasizing vegetables, while saving fruits and tubers to support intense exercise.

• Create an n-3/n-6 profile of 1:1 to 1:2 by eating predominately grass-fed meats and wild-caught fish, while limiting n-6 intake.

EIGHT

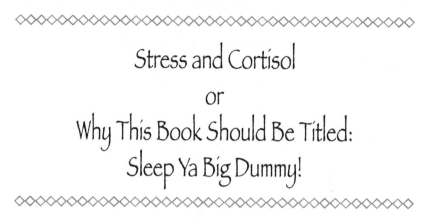

Introductions are always a bugger for me because I'm not a linear thinker. I see the world as layers of connections rather than some kind of university-style outline. This is great for making connections and innovation, but it's a terrible way to introduce new material to most people. If everything is connected, how do you keep the moving parts separated such that one can make heads or tails of the material?

This chapter is a perfect illustration of this challenge, as we begin to look more and more at an integrated approach to our Paleo Solution. We must consider more endocrinology, specifically the adrenal hormone cortisol and its many actions on both wellness and disease. Then we will explore how our modern lives are growing more and more at odds with our ancestral lifeway, and what this means not only for cortisol, but also for (you guessed it) our performance, health, and longevity.

It is this point of divergence from our ancestral lifeway—the separation of how our genetics expect to meet the world vs. how they actually *do* meet the world—that is the issue. If you want to understand how and why our modern world is killing us softly, you need to understand where we came from. Then, if you want to, you can affect change that complements our genetics and ancestry.

Way Back

It may test your credulity, but our ancestors had things both harder and easier than we do. Hard things included living without advances such as medicine, centralized government, or advanced communications. If you broke a leg, caught a nasty bug, or got mauled by a large, nasty critter—well, these types of things explain the average lifespan of about thirty to thirty-five years for our hunter-gatherer ancestors. As you will discover in the exercise chapter, our ancestors lived a rough and tumble existence that left their skeletons looking like equal parts Olympic athlete and rodeo clown!

Our forebears had to work quite hard for their food, clothing, and shelter, often at significant risk of bodily harm. Interestingly, however, they did not work as hard or as long as we do. It may come as a shock, but our ancestors only worked about 10–15 hours per week. Pause for a moment and let that sink in. Perhaps they worked five hours one day, a few hours the next. Then they took an entire day off to just laze about. This may seem impossible, but it is a common feature of *all* hunter-gatherer societies studied, and this is why the HG lifeway is often referred to as the "original affluent lifestyle."

Their work varied with the seasons and locations in which they lived. It provided food, clothing, and shelter. A hunter-gatherer's work also supplied the backbone of Paleo-insurance: a place in the extended family network of a hunter-gatherer tribe. The rest of the time was spent socializing, traveling to see relatives in neighboring groups, and oftentimes playing games of chance. Even cavemen liked to gamble!

Explorers and anthropologists who have studied and lived among various HG tribes describe the people as "very" content and happy. Early to bed, early to rise, and lots of adventure (a little danger can kill you, but oddly enough, it also lets you know you are alive). They had a strong social network, a sense of belonging, variety in their work and, really, not that much drudgery. Now I do not want to paint an overly beatific view of the HG life. They certainly faced a number of stressors: Sickness, injury, and perhaps attack by wild animal, a rival tribe, or even a relative (then, as now, the most likely person to kill you was someone you knew). Although these dangers might shatter the Walt

Disney utopia I was painting, our ancestors lived what appears to be remarkably good lives considering the lack of things like medicine, insulated homes, and sitcoms.

The key difference between the stressors our ancestors faced and our modern stressors can be described thusly: frequency and duration. Paleo stress tended to be acute: short in duration and infrequent in occurrence. Modern stress, by contrast, tends to be constant and unrelenting.

In the book, *Why Zebras Don't Get Ulcers*, Prof. Robert M. Sapolsky makes the point that wild animals do not show the stress-related illnesses we see in humans. Part of this is due to how the human condition has changed (Paleo vs. present life) and part of this is due to the nature of the human mind. Humans can fret about the future, and review unsettling memories of the past. Psychoneuroimmunology (how the mind influences the immune system and vice versa) has shown that our thoughts are our reality, for good or ill.

A theme Eastern religions share is a recommendation to "be in the now." Kids and other small scampering critters tend to be quite proficient at being present, and it's little wonder that we associate happiness with the simple lives of kids and critters. Modern life, for all its advances and amazing achievements, has opened its own Pandora's box. Unlike the story of Pandora, however, in which a host of demons have been set loose upon humanity, I think the analogy is that we have been thrown *into* the box and the stresses of modern life assail us from every angle.

I know, it's kinda heavy stuff. Here's the deal though: Until you can recognize the bars of your cage (or the walls of your box?), you do not stand a chance of getting out. In the words of Erwan Le Corre, founder of MovNat, you are a "Zoo Human." Ponder this image for a moment. It is both accurate and unpleasant. Hopefully the imagery motivates you to make some changes, or, again in Erwan's words, "to find your true nature."

With that in mind, let's look at modern life with the perspective that our genetics are wired for the acute stressors of the Paleolithic, and then let's see if we can formulate a plan of escape. I saw a few vegans up the street, maybe we can push them down, take their hemp, and "braid an escape rope!"

Modern Life—Sleep Much?

What better way to chronicle the stressors of modern life than to look at how we greet most days:

1. With an alarm clock.
2. Without as much sleep as we would like to have.

I'll talk about the physiology of sleep in a moment, but for now I think we can all agree that we feel dramatically better with sufficient sleep. Or, if you are like most people, you have no idea what "well rested" means. "Sleeping in" and being fully rested is our ancestral, genetic norm. Unfortunately, we rarely experience this after infancy. Well, not until we are pooping our pants in a rest home.

What would your life be like if you could awaken every day *without* an alarm and after sleeping as much as you wanted? This is *not* a rhetorical question. Contemplate.

Commute

How many of you walk or ride a bike to and from your work? Not bloody many, I'd wager. If you live in Europe or one of the few forward-thinking cities in America or Canada, you have some public transport options that afford some degree of relaxation (other than the threat of physical violence and mugging in the city, but we will overlook that for now). For many people, their daily commute can represent a long, frustrating process that looks nothing like gearing up for a hunting trip or a foray to collect edible plants. One of the key determinates for many people considering a career move or relocating the family is the effect commuting will have on one's quality of life. On the flip side of this are those folks who opt for a longer commute so they can make more money to have a bigger house and more crap.

Work

Do you *love* your work? Like it? Tolerate it for the sake of survival? Most people like what they do well enough, but frequently share the sentiment that they would like to do less of it. How many of you work forty hours per week? Fifty? More than this? Forty-hour work weeks are considered anemic by most standards; yet this represents two and a half to four times more time than our ancestors spent working. That is a big deal when we consider stress. Unlike our generalist ancestors, most of us focus on a specialty that becomes, quite literally, a grind. When viewed in this way, it makes sense why we are fired up for work on Monday and Tuesday, but looking up the number for the Hemlock Society on Thursday and Friday! This may not jibe with our Puritan work ethic, but we *might* be working more than is good for us. I don't want to make anyone uncomfortable (that's a lie, I am actually hoping to make you wickedly uncomfortable. I'd like to see you really give this stuff some thought), but if you have ever felt that working a little less and having more variety in your life would relieve stress and provide you with energy, you are likely correct.

Family and Social Life

Did you know people who lack supportive familial and social bonds are as at risk to develop illness or die as pack-a-day smokers? Why might that be? Well, because we evolved as social beings. We have considered a number of situations in which excess (carbohydrates, stress, work) has deleterious effects on health. Similarly, however, a deficiency can kill us just as dead. Such examples include sleep deprivation, inactivity, or inadequate social bonds. Few of us have social networks remotely on a par with that experienced by our ancestors, and this registers as a serious stress. Put the book down and go make a friend, OK?

Activity (You Know, Exercise)

We will look at a whole chapter on exercise, but I want to point out a few things: Our Paleolithic ancestors tended to be very active, but they also managed to get quite a bit of rest. On average, our ancestors hunted and gathered the energy equivalent of about 11 miles of walking per day. This activity was split among a multitude of tasks (there is that variety thing again). As a result of not being overly repetitive, their activity had less negative impact on their joints and minds.

Our modern life, by contrast, seems to deposit people into one of two camps.

1. Folks who are efficiency experts and endeavor to do as little as possible. Five steps from sofa to refrigerator, six steps to the car in the garage, twenty steps from parking space to work station. These people seriously consider a catheter to avoid the exertion of walking to the bathroom.

2. People who attempt suicide by exercise. Up at 4 AM six days per week. Run, bike, and swim, all before the rooster crows. Lift weights at lunch. Work out even when sick, bleeding, or delirious. I get tired even thinking about you people!

In the Paleo Solution, we shoot for a therapeutic dose of exercise. Enough to make sure your fanny is firm and scrumptious-looking and your blood lipids make your cardiologist sing with happiness, but not so much exercise that you burn yourself out and make a bad situation worse.

I think you have a basic idea about how our lifestyles might be a teensy bit out of balance relative to our cave dweller genetics. Sleep, activity, socialization, and meaningful work. Check! Now we need to look at what is going on inside. In good times and bad. We need to look closely at the hormone cortisol, and see how it fits into our Paleolithic Solution.

Cortisol

Without being the least bit cynical, I could boil life down to food, sleep, and sex.* On the food side of the equation, we have all that goes into getting it (brains to plan, brawn to procure and defend). Once we have that food, we eat it and either burn it or store it. This is all related to our short and long term energy management, body-fatness, fertility, etc. In-

---

*I have presented this as a generalization when, in fact, there is intraspecies variation on this topic. If you have the genetic markers "XY," everything in fact boils down to just sex. If you carry the "XX" genotype, things are significantly more complex. Food must be accompanied by a cacao derivative. Sleep requires some kind of garment, generally referred to as "PJs," and sex can be readily interchanged with social phenomena nearly fatal to the XYs of our species, "Romantic Comedies."

sulin and glucagon are there to help regulate our storage and utilization of energy. However, Cortisol is also a player in this game, as it also has effects on energy storage and a host of other functions:

1. Regulating the immune response. Too much of an immune response can lead to autoimmunity or significant problems from "collateral damage" caused by an overactive immune system. Many diseases are not fatal in and of themselves (like the H1N1 flu), but they sometimes become fatal because of an overreaction by the immune system. Cortisol "puts the breaks" on the immune system and is very important in both our susceptibility to disease and how we respond to illness.

2. How much sodium we have in our blood. More cortisol means more sodium and thus more blood volume. Typically, this will lead to higher blood pressure, with the associated stress on the heart, vasculature, and kidneys.

3. Regulates connective tissue strength. Too much cortisol can weaken connective tissue in our skin and elsewhere. Cortisol can and does make you wrinkle faster.

4. Perhaps most important to our discussion here, cortisol releases glucose and fatty acids from the liver and blunts insulin sensitivity.

Most people are familiar with the idea that cortisol is a "stress" hormone, but this is misleading and more a function of our modern lives than cortisol really being a "stress" hormone. Cortisol is in fact critical to life, and a lack of cortisol will mean significant health problems, including death! This is again a story of shooting for the right amount of a hormone, and if you have been paying attention thus far, we are talking about levels that we might find in our Paleolithic ancestors.

A normal day for our Paleolithic ancestors would start by awakening with relatively high cortisol levels. This is *not* the Monday morning commute blues: Paleo Edition. This is nature's way of making sure we are alert, energized, and ready to go! Cortisol causes the release of glucose and fatty acids from the liver. That's energy our Paleolithic ancestors needed to move camp, hunt, gather, and generally get the day

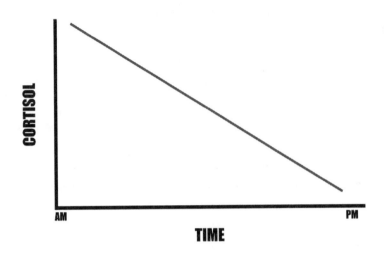

Normal cortisol profile. High in the AM, low in the PM.

going. Now, this scenario was normal and, in fact, *nonstressful*. Keep in mind there are normal operating parameters for all our hormones and it is quite normal for Cortisol to be elevated in the morning.

Cortisol works in synchrony with insulin and glucagon to regulate our energy levels. When we need more energy (early in the day or fleeing from a predator) Cortisol is relatively high. In the evening, when we are winding down and going to bed, Cortisol should drop. Now, what if our Paleolithic ancestors were ambushed by a rival camp or they stumbled upon a particularly large and cranky carnivore that wanted to see just who was at the top the food chain that day? Did those situations happen and were they stressful? Yes, they happened, and yes, they were stressful. But the stresses of Paleolithic consequence sorted themselves out quickly. For good or ill. They tended not to drag on and they did not happen every day.

Our modern life may not involve the risk of being eaten by a bear (generally), but it does come with a host of its own stressors. Some quite immediate and tangible, others more mental. But in general, our stressors in modern times are chronic, as opposed to the acute stresses for which we are so well equipped. Possibly losing a job in a bad economy, getting mugged while on the train, a near miss while driving, thinking about the kids' college education . . . *lack of sleep*. These are modern issues that register as a stress, and in a cumulative fashion, they can crush us.

Beat That Dead Horse White Boy!

The critical concept here is acute vs. chronic stress. We are genetically wired for dealing with acute (brief/infrequent) stress. This stress was answered with some kind of physical activity (fight or flight) that made use of that glucose and fat released from the liver. Then things returned to a relatively "mellow" norm.

We are not well suited to the stresses of modern life. These stresses affect people in different ways and to different degrees, but they are most assuredly "there," and they are cumulative.

When you are subjected to stress, particularly chronic stress, your body releases cortisol much more frequently than it should. This gets ugly when cortisol is not only high in the morning, but all day long, even at bedtime. The consequences can be dire, as the more stressed we get, the worse our ability to deal with stress becomes. It is a nasty snowball effect that is called a "feed forward" mechanism in biology. Abnormally elevated cortisol begins to disturb sleep, which makes us more prone to daily stress, which raises cortisol. The consequences of this downward spiral include suppressed immune function, chronically elevated blood sugar levels, decreased insulin sensitivity, impaired ability to form long-term memory, and decreased sex drive and libido. Yes folks, cortisol is a big deal.

You Know . . . Everything Is Like Related. And Stuff.

Chronic stress can and does raise cortisol levels. Stress can come from a variety of places and is somewhat subjective, but one of the first things to be affected by stress and increased cortisol is sleep. Once your sleep gets buggered, the wheels fall off the wagon. Keep in mind this works both ways. An otherwise manageable stress level can be made nearly fatal by sleep disturbances. Staying up too late, or simply neglecting sleep quality and duration, can seriously undermine your ability to deal with otherwise manageable levels of stress.

I Make Sleepy Time

Most people realize they feel subpar when they miss sleep. Other people are so consistently sleep deprived they have no idea what normal is. Wherever you are on that spectrum, you need a wake-up call on beddy-bye. Why? Well, here are two biggies: Just one night of missed or inadequate sleep is sufficient to make you as insulin resistant as a type 2 diabetic. Think about how crappy you feel when you miss sleep. That's how much fun it is to be a type 2 diabetic all the time! Exercise can help, but your physiology never gets to normal without adequate sleep.

I can hear the tough guys and gals out there, "Sleep's a crutch; it's all in the mind. I'm tough; I just need more coffee and I can push through." Uh, sure, tough guy, how about this: The Centers for Disease Control recently announced that shift work (aka—lack of sleep) is a known carcinogen. Billy-Bob that means shift work, similar to cigarettes, asbestos, nuclear radiation, and certain talk shows can give you cancer. OK, maybe I'm stretching things on the talk shows. When you neglect sleep or have poor sleep quality, this registers as a significant stressor to your body. It makes you immune compromised, chubby, forgetful, and crazy.

Our hunter-gatherer ancestors never had an alarm clock. They went to bed when the sun went down (or not long thereafter) and got up when the sun came up. Our ancestors, like every other living thing, were tuned to the ebb and flow of not only the seasons, but also the turning of the day. It was not "24/7" as we live now. As I described earlier, we had significant periods of leisure and downtime, and we *slept*. This is what our genetics are expecting when we are born into this world, but we are now sending a very different message. If your genetics could talk to you, they would likely take on the voice of Bill Cosby and say, "I brought you into this world . . . I can take you out!"

But Robb, I Just Want to Look Good!

If the notion of cancer caused by lack of sleep is not motivational to you, I'll go for a more superficial shot—How about looking good naked. Interested yet? If you do not sleep you will:

1. Completely cock-block your fat loss.
2. Get fat, sick, and diabetic.
3. Get old and wrinkled before your time.

If we are chronically insulin resistant and have elevated blood glucose levels from cortisol, it is quite similar to eating a high-carb diet. Advanced glycation end-products age our skin and organs at an accelerated rate. Insulin resistance causes us to store fat around the waistline and we tend to not use body fat for energy. Additionally, elevated cortisol destabilizes the protein collagen, which is what gives youthful skin its, well, youthfulness!

Even if your food is pretty good, you can undermine your health (and fanny) by mismanagement of stress and sleep. So, for those of you who choose to stick your collective heads in the sand on the health issues, perhaps you are superficial enough to do something to avoid getting fat, wrinkled, and diabetic. I don't really care what your motivation is—I just want you to give this stuff a shot so you can see how effective it is. Oh, and your fanny looks a lot better if it's not droopy and wrinkled!

Let's Talk about Charlie

Here is a hypothetical example of how stress can accumulate in our lives. Charlie is a composite of thousands of people I have worked with. In fact, Charlie might be you.

Charlie has a great job, which is fantastic because he knows many people that have been laid off. Charlie is working extra hard to prove his worth to his company and because he has a beautiful six-month-old daughter. Charlie likes to stay in shape. Not only does exercise make him feel good, but his job has a "meet-and-greet" component, so if he is fit and attractive, he is better at his job. Charlie found a new high-intensity interval training program that he does five days per week. The only class he can make is at 6 AM, so he gets up at 4:30 every day to make it to the gym. When he gets home, he helps his wife before heading off to work.

As of late, Charlie has noticed little "pop" in his exercise, and although he is watching his food tighter than ever, he seems to be getting soft in the abs. He *always* had a six-pack, but now he is flabby in the gut. Although he rarely caves and eats something he should not, he has been dealing with wicked sugar cravings in the afternoons and evenings. He's had difficulty concentrating in a number of circumstances—at work, while driving, and even at home. This is not like him at all, as he is usually the guy who remembers "everything," whether related to work or pop-culture quizzes on the radio.

All Charlie wants to do is sleep, but when he puts his head down at night, his mind races. He does not get to bed till 10:00 or 10:30, and it is another hour or longer before he falls asleep most nights. He frequently awakes around 3:30 needing to pee (when did that start happening?). When his alarm jangles him awake, he feels more tired than when he went to bed! Charlie always thinks to himself upon waking, "Why can't I be this tired when I go to sleep"?

Some days are worse than others. Last Tuesday, he nearly spilled the shake he was drinking while driving to the gym. Once at the gym, he felt achy and cold. For the first time in his life, he felt old. Instead of feeling thirty-five, he felt eighty. To make matters worse, he had another tickle in his throat—most likely another sinus infection. He death-marched through that day like all the rest, and even forgot an important meeting (having neglected to get that scheduled into his PDA—he *never* used to miss details like that!).

When he arrived home that Tuesday evening at 6 PM, he grabbed his cooing six-month-old daughter from his wife so she could finish dinner. His wife enjoyed being at home with their new daughter, but she was a night-shift nurse, and in a few weeks she would be heading back to work. Working back-to-back shifts was no picnic, but her supplemental income was the only way they could afford the beautiful new townhouse they had purchased eighteen months prior.

After dinner, Charlie and his wife had a rare moment alone as their daughter slept in the living room. Charlie's wife, half jokingly, half scolding, pointed out that Charlie had not "made a move on her" since their daughter was born. Charlie felt guilty. He deeply loved his wife, but he had been far more interested in sleeping than sex as of late.

Analyzing Charlie

I have worked with many "Charlies" over the past ten years. Sometimes it's Charlene instead of Charlie, but the net result is the same, as is the cause: a lifestyle completely out of whack with our genetics.

Let's dissect the stressors to understand what is happening to Charlie's health and hormonal status. Keep in mind: Charlie is doing a lot of stuff right. Exercising, watching his food, staying in a loving and supportive relationship. Think about how things might go if his food was terrible, he never exercised, and had relationship problems. I've worked with that person a few thousand times too, and it's an even worse train wreck.

Sleep

How much is Charlie getting? Not remotely enough. He is getting into bed about 10:30, is awake for an hour or so after that, and then get's up in the night to pee. He's up at 4:30, resulting in less than six hours most nights, perhaps as little as four to four and a half when considering his potty breaks.

Tired and Wired

If you recall, Charlie is dragging-fanny through the day. Barely able to stay awake, forgetful. When he lies down to sleep, his head spins as he reviews the day's events and thinks about the following day's activities. Charlie is what strength coach Charles Poliquin would call "tired and wired." Normally, our cortisol is low at night to allow us to go to sleep. In Charlie's case, he is in a stage of burnout in which his cortisol is actually high in the evening and rock bottom in the morning. This makes life particularly tough, as the little rest he gets is not all that restful, and when he needs to be "on," he is anything but.

A common solution to this problem is downers at night and uppers in the AM. Downers usually entail a few glasses of wine (It helps Charlie "relax") and an ever-increasing dose of coffee in the morning. The problem is the wine makes that disturbed sleep even worse because it blocks the critical release of growth hormone in early sleep. The escalating morning stimulant dose helps initially, but it just digs a deeper

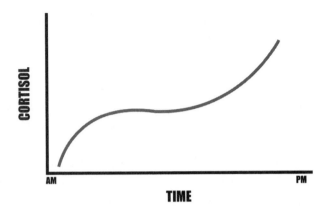

Tired and wired profile: Low cortisol in the Am, high in the PM.

hole in the long run. At some point, the coffee no longer provides any noticeable boost—it is simply vital to existence. Functioning without it is not even an option.

Some people will take the "uppers and downers" game to their family physician. He or she will prescribe one of a variety of sleep aids, which again blocks growth hormone release (your rest is just not that restful on drugs, folks) and the uppers may shift to things like Ritalin from a coworker. The bottom line is Charlie is *not* getting enough sleep and the pharmaceutical routes only delay the inevitable and worsen the fall.

Sporting a Chubby

Charlie, although not fat by most people's standards, is fatter than he has ever been in his life. He battles his newly acquired sweet-tooth and constantly works out, but what the heck is happening?

Charlie has chronically elevated cortisol levels, which means chronically elevated blood sugar (released from the liver) and fatty acid levels. This indirectly impairs insulin sensitivity (from the high blood sugar), while cortisol directly inhibits insulin sensitivity and leptin sensitivity. It's a classic sign of insulin-resistant fat storage, which is why Charlie gains weight around the midsection. If we look at Charlie's blood lipids, we would see his triglycerides inching up, likely in lockstep with his LDL count, while the particle size becomes small, dense, and reactive. Atherosclerosis anyone?

Sex Type Thing

Charlie has two new, but very annoying things happening. Low sex drive and a need to pee at night. As Charlie's body fat increases, he has a tendency to convert his meager testosterone into estrogen because of an enzyme called aromatase that hangs out in fat tissue. If your body fat increases, whether male or female, you tend to convert testosterone to estrogen. For Charlie, this has set in motion prostate growth (benign prostatic hyperplasia—BPH) at the ripe old age of thirty-five. If this was not bad enough, his testosterone levels are low for two reasons. Cortisol and testosterone compete for the same limited resources. If cortisol goes up, testosterone *must* go down. Then add the conversion of testosterone to estrogen due to increased body fat and we have a bad situation brewing for Charlie. The effects for women are similarly powerful with a tendency to produce PMS, PCOS, fibroids, and infertility. Fun, no?

Did You Say Something?

Memory, from a biological perspective, falls into two categories: Necessary for survival or "quaint and expendable." High cortisol levels make memories "quaint" because your body thinks it is in a fight to the death. In most fight-to-the-death scenarios, you will remember enough of that event to avoid it in the future (hopefully), but there is no need to imprint languages, mathematics, or silly things like that. High cortisol not only blocks new memories, it actually causes some of our most valuable gray matter to *die*. Yes, a T-shirt with the slogan, "Cortisol causes brain damage" would not be lying. Now, you might be inclined to dismiss most of this stuff, but the combined features of insulin resistance and oxidative stress characteristic of high cortisol levels are in fact eerily similar to the proposed mechanisms of fun things like Parkinson's, Alzheimer's, and dementia. I guess the one upside of losing your marbles is that every time you see your significant other it will literally be like the first time: "Hey, Sexy! What's your name?"

Stressed Much?

Charlie has a ton of stress from which he cannot escape, but he is actually pretty mellow by disposition. Are you like Charlie, or do you have

significant conflict in your life? Are you wound tight, and do you have
constant emotional ups and downs? If your answers are yes, you likely
have impaired insulin sensitivity. Now your behavior could actually
be *from* poor insulin sensitivity due to bad diet and inadequate sleep
(remember how it feels to crash from too many carbs?), but it could be
that your stress is actually *causing* your insulin resistance. As I mentioned in the previous section, when we are subjected to stress for a
long period of time, our body will tend to produce too much cortisol.
Cortisol is helpful in stressful situations (from a Paleolithic perspective), as it releases stored energy from the liver in the form of glucose
and fats. When running from a bear, this is a good thing. In today's
world, however, your stressed-out hissy fit is pretty similar to eating a
candy bar, but without any of the fun. You release sugar and fats from
your liver because your genetics think you are in danger, and you may
need to run or fight for your life. Instead you are overrun by stress and
your health and waistline are paying the price. Just to be clear: You
could be eating a smart, low-carb, Paleo diet, and still fail to see many
benefits due to chronically high stress.

Recap Numero Dos

Buttercup, I think you missed some of that due to impaired concentration caused by lack of sleep and excessive stress. Let's make sure you
got everything:

Stress has an additive effect. We lose some sleep, work longer hours,
fret about money, and take care of the kids. Each of these adds to our
stress buffet. Sleep is likely the most important factor (neglect your
sleep and watch how fast things come undone) concerning stress, but
day-to-day stress can elevate cortisol in the evening and leave you tired
and wired, thus affecting sleep. It's a catch-22 if you don't have your
ducks in a row. Meds and booze do not fix the situation. Any questions?

Your Fix
So, I guess it would be mean to get you all worked up about stress and
cortisol and then offer no solutions.

Being the consummate professional, I'm going to walk you through the most important things you need to do to get a handle on your stress. A few of you who are *really* sick may need to take this a step further and seek some medical help for adrenal glands that are "high mileage." Some of you are in the midst of chronically elevated cortisol, but you can save your own bacon *if* you start making some changes. To be successful we need to bring your stress and cortisol back into ancestral norms.

Dude, Rack Out

It might be important to know how much sleep is enough: for most people, most of the time, eight to nine and a half hours per night. For some of you that is legitimately too much—you just need to awaken refreshed and *sans alarm clock*. No ringy-dingy! If you have historically gotten by with six or seven hours and you seem fine, good on ya, but you need one little tweak to that formula: your bedroom must be pitch black when you sleep. That seems pretty self-explanatory, but I'll spell it out: no light sources! No TVs, computers, or alarm clocks. Fire alarms need to have their lights covered. A sleep mask does not cut it. If you want all the details of why, read the excellent book *Lights Out! Sleep, Sugar and Survival*. The abbreviated story goes like this: the porphyrin proteins that make up your red blood cells register light and carry this information of light exposure to your brain. This information blocks a very important antioxidant hormone/neurotransmitter called melatonin. This process is at the heart of your problem with cortisol. So get black-out curtains and cover your light sources to ensure a deep, restful sleep. Capisce?

This goes for everyone, but I know some of you will be incredulous about this. I have worked with many people who swore they only needed to sleep six or seven hours per night. These same people, when they slept in a completely dark environment, suddenly added an hour or two to that sleep and, miraculously, they looked, felt, and performed better!

If you get a handle on your sleep, you will recover faster from exercise, have better memory and recall, and have fewer allergies and significantly less inflammation. All of the stuff we talked about with

regards to insulin and inflammation, sleep affects this about as powerfully as food.

If you are sick or overweight, this is a nonnegotiable topic. Para-
phrasing a line from the book *Lights Out:* Sleeping more might cut
into your social life, but so will cancer, diabetes, and dementia! Just to
further guilt you into this, you have already bought, stole, or borrowed
this book. Your investment is already done. What do you think my motivation is in recommending this stuff? Oddly, my desire is to see you
succeed. I do not have a "Robb Wolf Sleep in a Box" product for sale.
This stuff works, but only if you *do* it. Oh yea, take the night-light out
of your kids' rooms. They will be pissed if they realize you are trying
to give them cancer and diabetes.

Shift Work

Do you work in police, military, fire, or medical service? If so, shift
work is likely a part of your gig. Well, you need to do the best you can
with this. You are not on an ideal schedule, but when you *do* sleep, it
needs to be quality. Dark room, full duration—it's tough, but it's critical. Naps help for folks in this situation but it is *not* a replacement for
full, restful sleep. Sorry.

Activity

Let's talk a little bit about "activity." I could have used the word "exercise," but activity sounds more sophisticated and won't cause you
to inch toward the door. I'm only going to touch on this briefly, as we
will have a whole chapter to bore you with later. For now, I just want to
throw out some general concepts.

The Paleo Solution shoots for a variety of exercise: a little some
days, a lot others, and occasionally none at all. Just like our hunter-
gatherer ancestors. Some of you have already given yourselves a "gold
star" for working out twice per day for the past five years. You're so
dedicated you even work out while sick! Yippee! Well, no gold star for
you! You are at the other end of the extreme and need to calm down.
We are trying to reduce stress and cortisol. In our gym we see people,
usually the endurance types, who seriously overdo their training. Are
you carrying some excess chub around the midsection despite "tons of

cardio"? Well Buttercup, all that cardio and getting up early to train has released more than your fair share of cortisol. And it's made you fat.

We see this routinely: Someone has been training with us for a year or so, has gotten quite lean and strong, and now he or she wants to tackle a marathon. Or a triathlon. Training volume goes from three days per week to six, and oddly the individual gets chubby in the midsection. Honestly, I don't care what you do, but if you think more, more, more is better, better, better, you are wrong. In the exercise chapter we will figure out what is a good dose to keep you lean, strong, and healthy.

I Like the Nightlife! I've Got to Boogie!

Ahhh, booze! So much fun, such a great way to ruin your health! Here is how most folks try to live: Stay up late watching TV and checking Facebook updates. Then head out on the town to shake your groove thang because you owe it to yourself to blow off some steam! Yeah, baby! You work hard so you deserve to play hard! Oh man! Everything is getting sooo hard around here! Wooohoo! That's the advertising fantasy of amazing nights of gin-soaked excitement. The cortisol-steeped reality is a shitty bar, creepy people, expensive booze, and a morning wakeup that feels like a breakfast date with the county coroner.

For our clients the lifestyle piece is tougher to nail down than the exercise for sure, and it is even tougher than the food. People will gladly pay to be beaten senseless in workouts, but they are ready to bolt when we suggest they get a few zzz's and curtail their boozing for the sake of their health and a better-looking fanny.

Other people find compliance difficult due to the nature of their work. Our realtors, for example, are socialites whose productivity is based on shaking hands, kissing babies, and drinking eight nights out of seven. I'm not a teetotaler myself, and I do not recommend that for you, but some common sense is in order here. I cannot tell you how many people have e-mailed or asked during seminars how to drink like they are "Leaving Las Vegas," yet remain lean and healthy. I'm honestly stupefied by some of the questions I get, as a little common sense will get you a long way!

It might in fact be necessary to cut back your boozing if you want to be leaner and healthier. I know it sounds ridiculous to some of you, but people ask this *all the time*. I think you can reasonably have a drink (perhaps two) a few nights per week and be fine. If you are sick and overweight, you do not have as much latitude (are you picking up on the theme here?). Now, all that considered, there are smarter and dumber ways to get your booze on. Here are field-tested booze recommendations from a biochemistry graduate from America's top party school:

Happy Hour

Alcohol has a nasty effect on dating standards and growth hormone release. It is outside the scope of this book to address your beer goggles, so we will stick with the purely physiological ramifications of alcohol consumption. What you need to know is that alcohol does not just blunt growth hormone release, it just turns it off. This is *not* good for your health, recovery, or body composition. Solution? Well, I'd *never* want to make you uncomfortable and suggest perhaps not being a lush . . . so here is what we do: Drink earlier. You need to get your booze in as far away from bedtime as you can. I will not give you liver clearance rates of alcohol so you can try to figure out how to "beat the system." You just need to get your main drinking done earlier in the evening.

In the Clear

Much of the problem with drinking is not the booze itself but all the crap, usually sugar, that comes along with it. Ditch your froufrou drinks with the umbrellas and go for clear liquor. My favorite is Tequila (gold), prepared with the following ingredients:

The Infamous NorCal Margarita!
2 shots of gold tequila
Juice of 1 lime (the whole damn thing!)
Splash of soda water.

Drink one or two of these on an empty stomach *early* in your evening. Wrap up the night with some protein and fat, and you are set. You socialized, got your head change, and did not do too much damage to yourself. There is also some chemistry behind the recommendations. The lime juice blunts insulin release and the carbon dioxide bubbles in the soda water act as what's called a "nonpolar solvent." This actually extracts the alcohol from the drink and delivers it to your system faster. Better living through chemistry!

Can you use another clear alcohol besides Tequila?
Yes, none are as good, but use whatever you like.

What about beer and wine?
Beer is generally loaded with gluten. If you can find a gluten-free variety, give it a shot, but keep in mind it does have significant sugar content. As to wine, I detest the stuff and think it had its best day when it was still grape juice. If you go for wine, opt for dry varieties, as they have less sugar. If you think you are drinking wine "for your health," this is as shaky an excuse as explaining away an adulterous liaison as "networking." In both situations, you are fooling no one but yourself.

But alcohol isn't *Paleo*! Why are you recommending this?
Because, I get this question every damn day and I'm just providing the information necessary to help people make the best choice for their situation. Let's not turn this into a religion, OK?

Neolithic Foods

Remember that chapter on grains, legumes, and dairy? Remember how that stuff is really damaging to your innards and can cause a ton of problems? Yeah, it gets worse. Those foods also release cortisol. Many people who have food intolerances will notice an increased pulse rate after eating that food. If these foods are damaging the gut (and they are), it registers as a stress on the body, and the response to stress is cortisol. This situation is not a one-way street by the way. Let's say you tolerate grains relatively well (at least better than I do, as even a tiny gluten exposure will lay me up for days). What if you were suddenly exposed to a significant stress? You had to care for an ailing parent, you had to work a huge amount of overtime at work, your sleep gets seriously impacted, you are pushing too hard getting ready for your marathon. How do you think this stress might affect your tolerance to Neolithic foods like grains, legumes, and dairy? Interestingly enough, this life stress has a very negative impact on your gut health, which then has an impact on your ability to deal with that stress, which can then impact your sleep. It all fits together.

Do You Own Your Things, or Do Your Things Own You?

My background is that of a scientist, athlete, and coach. In many ways, you could order out a person's thinking in those different areas from concrete to very fluid and instinctual. Chemistry certainly benefits from intuition and insight, but it is 90 percent information and analysis and 10 percent intuition (I'm just making these numbers up, walk with me on this). On the other side, coaching is best when the coach has a solid technical basis and then he or she goes on a gestalt-like instinct. Perhaps 10 percent science, 90 percent intuition. Well, this next piece comes more from the perspective of a coach. I should probably say "life coach," but that term creeps me out for some reason. I will try to bring in a little science in the form of some psychology and anthropology to support my pending statement, but this is much more a felt thing, and I want you to take it from that context.

Ok, here it is: Having more shit (cars, TVs, houses, shoes . . . you know, crap) does *not* make you happier. In fact, it makes you unhappy and whittles away your life and causes you stress.

Ok, it's out. Now let's look at this. I am a dyed-in-the wool libertarian. I love free markets, business, and freedom. I also think people get easily swayed into thinking a big house, fast car, or the latest gadgets, will make them happy. I see people doing more work than they want so they can buy crap they worry about and must maintain. We have a client who bought a very expensive car. She has the money, and has worked hard her whole life, so I certainly believe she should do whatever she wants to do to make herself happy. But now all she does is complain about how people cut her off in traffic, make dirty faces at her, and how much stress it is to park and maintain this high-dollar car. Now this client, who is a wonderful person, is really overweight and not really happy in her own skin. She has worked so hard for so long, only to be stressed about her big house and expensive car. She has been the epitome of stress for twenty years and has an autoimmune condition, cardiovascular disease, and obesity for her reward. As she slowly regains her health, she is realizing time, health, and experiences are what matter, not a remodel on a house that was new two years ago. Her illness is largely an outgrowth of the stress necessary to maintain the stuff in her life.

Another example is a young couple that have good-paying jobs, two kids, and so much stress they want to run away. Their issue? During the housing boom they bought as much fracking house as they could. They, like many other people, were banking on the house appreciating, so why not swing for the fences and get as much as they could? They also made sure to appoint their house with all new furniture, a big TV, and new cars for mama-bear and papa-bear. The only problem with this all-too-typical American dream is they never really added up all of the individually small costs, and suddenly they were seriously over their heads. These folks are crushed by stress born of poor financial choices. These choices are driven by one of two compulsions: Trying to fill a void that tangible items will never fill, or by ego: *I want more stuff so people will respect me.*

These two stories are related in that they describe a serious mismatch between elements of our economy and our psychology. Credit is such a dicey thing for people because it is a completely novel concept in nature. You *never* get "something for nothing" in a living biological system. We never sauntered across the savannah and bought food, booze, and furniture on credit. There were no "deferred payments." You wanted something, you had to work to get it, and you experienced the full impact of that want immediately. Then you had the item, whether it was food, clothing, or shelter. But in a nomadic, hunter-gatherer society, you do not need or want that much stuff. If you needed something, you generally had the skills to make it. And unless it was critical, you damn sure did not want to lug it around with you!

I hesitated about even broaching this topic, as it is certainly "soft science." In my experience of working with people, stress is an inescapable and significant factor in people's lives, and a stunning amount of their stress is self-induced. People might benefit from considering how they want to spend their time and resources. I know wealthy people who use their wealth to live a fun, action-packed life (or a quiet contemplative life in some instances), but these people have remarkably little stuff as compared to their wealth. I see other folks who are payment-planned and stressed to the gills despite six- or seven-figure incomes.

To some degree I really buy into the idea that "attachment is suffering." If you are attached to a bunch of crap that requires you to work ungodly hours to pay for it, you are missing something. I also know people who *love* to work. They do not have an off switch and just love to go. If this is you, and you're happy, fulfilled, and satisfied, great. You are a rare breed indeed.

I'm not a guru, and I have no special knowledge. But I have seen a lot of people benefit from assessing what is important in their lives and making changes to support happiness. It's hard to do. We can make excuses about obligations and kids and all kinds of stuff. I don't know what the right answer is for *you*, but if you have weight or health issues, work yourself to death, have a closet full of clothes you never wear, and a house full of crap you never use, then maybe you need to do some thinking about how you approach your life.

I bring all this up because issues of materialism, happiness, credit, and work are talked about quite often, but I have never seen anyone turn an evolutionary light on this topic. Why is credit a tough concept to navigate? Because it's a novel concept that has some addictive characteristics, just like refined foods. Why do people spend their money (time) on duplicates of crap they do not need? Because it spins the same dials in our heads as hunting and gathering, only we have to lug the crap around with us now. Alcoholism, drug addiction, spending problems, and gambling tend to run in the same folks. We all have these tendencies to some degree, as they are all symptoms of an environment at odds with our genetics.

What about Me?

So, where are you with regards to cortisol, and health? How much do you have in common with Charlie described at the start of the chapter? Let's look at some specifics:

1. Do you sleep less than nine hours per night?
2. Do you have problems falling asleep or staying asleep?

3. Do you wake up more exhausted than when you went to bed?

4. Do you get a "second wind" in the evening, and really only feel awake about the time you *should* go to bed?

5. Are you tired and achy all the time?

6. Do you suffer frequent upper-respiratory infections?

7. Do you work out to exhaustion, and do you crave the "boost" exercise provides?

8. Do you live and die by stimulants such as coffee?

9. Have you gained fat in the midsection, despite watching your food intake?

10. Have you experienced memory problems?

11. Do you have problems with depression or seasonal affective disorder?

12. Do you remember what sex is?

At some point this list starts looking more like a horoscope than legitimate health information, but the reality is that elevated cortisol levels affect any system you can imagine. Body fat, cognition, fertility, exercise performance, immunity. What else is there? If you want to get more clinical in your investigations, you can ask your doctor to run an adrenal stress index (ASI). Hypercorticism (high cortisol levels) can cause problems with normal thyroid function, often contributing to hyper (elevated) thyroid.

The problem I've seen people face when dealing with this situation, myself included, is that our whole life contributes to the issue. People tend to change things enough to feel a little better, then slide back into old habits. If this is really an issue for you, it will take some trial and error to figure out how to make things work. Don't worry, you can do it. Your health, and your fanny, will thank you!

By the way, I noticed your sweatband and leg warmers. Must be time to work out.

NINE

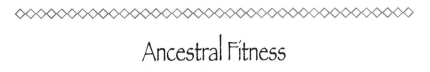

Ancestral Fitness

Every time I feel the urge to exercise, I sit down until it goes away.
—Mark Twain

If you work in sales or marketing, you are likely aware of the difference between features and benefits. A clock on your heating and air conditioning is a feature. Having a cozy, temperature-controlled house is the benefit. A steel toe with reinforced, triple-stitched leather are features of a work-boot. Not losing your toes if something heavy falls on them is the benefit!

People are usually motivated by benefits, and I have been contemplating how to sell you on the benefits of exercise, but for some reason, this just does not seem right. Do I want you to understand the importance of exercise and actually *do* some? Hell + Yes. But that does not seem enough. I do not want to cheapen this message, and I do not want to default into scare tactics because, Buttercup, it all boils down to this: If you do not exercise, you are broken.

Broken? Like . . . not OK? Not Whole? Incomplete?

Yes, correct on all counts.

Is this some kind of value judgment about you as a person? Am I trying to be mean? No, this is no value judgment, and no, I'm not trying to be mean. I'm just sharing a very important fact. Exercise is integral to you being who you are *meant* to be.

Whoa Robb! Are you getting metaphysical here?! Some kind of existentialist determinism?

No, that's not it at all . . . here's the deal:

You are born into this world with a set of genetics, half from Mum, half from Pops. Those genes are expecting you to run, jump, throw, tumble, dance, fight, flee, stalk, carry, build, wrestle, stroll, climb, drag, hike, sprint. You are meant to be active. *Really* active. There are few critters on this planet that do not expend significant energy finding food, avoiding danger, or looking for a mate. Well, except us. We can literally do almost nothing physical yet have food, clothing, shelter, and safety. This is fantastic in many ways, as living wild in nature has its pitfalls, but being sedentary can kill us just as surely as beast or foe. Don't believe me? The Centers for Disease Control list inactivity as the third leading cause of preventable death in the United States. Add poor diet to that, and we have the second leading cause, behind only tobacco. Cancer, neurodegeneration, diabetes, depression, frailty, loss in general capacity—all these and many other ills await the couch-bound.

How can this be?

Why does exercise matter so much?

Our hunter-gatherer ancestors lived an active and vigorous life. They and their prehuman ancestors had to expend remarkable amounts of energy to provide food, clothing, and shelter. Over the course of millions of years our genetics were forged with a level of activity not dissimilar from that of an Olympic caliber athlete. This is what our genetics are expecting when we are born into the world. We are literally "born to be fit." An unfortunate side effect of technology and affluence is the physical activity that made our ancestors strong and healthy is all but missing from our sedentary existences.

Micro-Mini-Me

On a molecular level this lack of exercise literally changes who we are. I can use a piece of technology called a microarray (a microchip with DNA attached to its surface), and I can "map" what genes are turned on or off in a person at a given time. Genetically speaking, this is "who you are," and it represents what is called your phenotype. Your geno-type is the mixed bag of genetics you received from Mum and Pops. Your phenotype is how those genetics are expressed.

How your genes experience the world (be it food, sleep, commu-nity, or exercise) influences how those genes are turned on or off and this determines your phenotype. So, I can take a microarray analysis of "Sedentary You" and analyze it for disease potential. If we then put you on a smart exercise program and look at how your genetics are expressing themselves in a few months, we will find that "Active You" is quite different from "Sedentary You." How different? It would be as if we were comparing your genetics with that of a random person off the street.

You are literally a different person when you exercise vs. when you do not.

Different how exactly?

Well, to fully understand that, and how valuable exercise is to you, we need to look at our ancestors and contemporary hunter-gatherers. Once we understand the amounts and types of exercise we are meant to do, we can do something about replicating this in our own lives. For those of you who are motivated by shiny objects, all you need to remember is, "if you exercise you will look good naked!"

Speaker for the Dead

One can learn a remarkable amount from a skeleton. Although bones, especially the sun-bleached variety, appear to be hard and static, living bones are highly plastic and reflect the environment to which they are exposed. If an arm is immobilized in a cast, we can see a remarkable decrease not only in muscle mass after a few weeks of disuse, but also a substantial decrease in the thickness of the arm bones themselves. This weakened state is reversed once normal activity is resumed for a few weeks. The stress of use increases both muscle size and the density of the underlying bone, which is an example of epigenetics: how the tissues of the arm alter their genetic expression as the environment is changed. We can see this in the difference between one hand and the other when we examine the muscle thickness and bone strength of an individual. Someone who is right handed will typically show significantly more muscular development, thickness of the points of attachment of the muscles to the bone, and the thickness and morphology of the bones themselves. Why? Because right-handers typically use their right hand more, subjecting that tissue to a greater load, which necessitates the adaptation of stronger muscles and bones.

This difference in bone thickness and morphology (how the bone is shaped) is largely dependent on the amounts and types of activity one is subjected to. The changes in bone structure can be quite rapid (as evidenced with an arm immobilized in a cast), and are very descriptive of the environment to which an organism lives.

The bones of our Paleolithic ancestors look like those of high-level athletes. Both have bones that are dense (high in mineral content) and show a structurally sound morphology or shape. Bone is not only strong due to the material from which it is made, but also because of the orientation of the growing, living crystal of the bone. Imagine chicken or duck eggs, which are remarkably strong when compressed from the outside, yet fragile enough for a baby chick to emerge when pushing from the inside. Bone that is heavily loaded is not only thicker, but it also shows an increased volume, which improves its strength and stability.

H. Erectus and *H. Neanderthalensis* skeletons show a level of activity and muscular development seen in only the most elite athletes of today. Early *H. Sapiens* showed a similar degree of development until about 40,000 years ago when several technological and social innovations improved the foraging techniques of our ancestors. These improvements are evidenced by more sophisticated weapons and tools in the archeological record, as well as a concomitant decrease in the physical development of the tool users. Although these Late Paleolithic ancestors were still very fit, strong, and active, especially by today's standards, the change in technology that improved the efficiency of hunting is clearly seen in the change in their less robust skeletal development.

Cross-training: Paleo Style

Although we can learn a remarkable amount about the fitness of hunter-gatherers from skeletons and archeological findings, nothing beats the real thing. When contemporary hunter-gatherers have been tested for strength, flexibility, and aerobic capacity, they have scored as well as highly trained athletes. No gyms, no physical education—simply living the active life that typifies the hunter-gatherer life-way.

From the !Kung of sub-Saharan Africa to the Ache of Peru, the foraging lifestyle necessitated the equivalent of fifteen to nineteen miles of walking—per day! This activity was devoted to a number of tasks and activities including hunting, collecting firewood and water, gathering plants and small animals, fishing, and traveling to see relatives. Some days were very intense and demanding, while other days were relaxed and might involve almost no activity beyond hanging out in camp.

This natural variability is likely woven into our genetics and explains both the benefit of cross-training (doing more than one activity to develop our fitness) and periodization (planned changes in exercise to avoid burnout and foster progress).

The foraging lifestyle left our ancestors lean, strong, and healthy. As we have talked about previously, although the life expectancy of HGs was relatively short due to illness and injury, those who lived into advanced age appear to have aged quite differently than most of us. They did not lose muscle mass or gain body fat as they aged. Decreases in flexibility were minimal, while certain inescapable elements of aging such as vision and hearing loss appear to have progressed at a much slower rate. By this point, you should recognize much of what passes for modern aging is simply a lifestyle at odds with our Paleolithic genes. How our HG counterparts lived and ate dramatically changed how they aged.

Muscles and Hormones

It appears the default mode for our species is the physique of a decathlete. Lean, muscled, and prepared for almost anything nature can unleash. We know this to be true based on the observations of modern HGs and the anthropological evidence: Thick, strong bones and muscle insertions typical of a hard-working athlete. The bones are evidence of relatively large, strong muscles, but what significance did this muscle play in the health of our ancestors, and presumably us?

Our muscle mass is some of the most metabolically active tissue in our bodies. When people talk about their "metabolism," it is not some weird item in their socks or in their armpit—it is their muscles! You may not think about muscle as being "healthy," but your level of muscularity is inversely proportional to your likelihood of dying. Starvation and advanced stages of AIDS share the feature that they become fatal once a certain threshold is passed in which an individual loses too much muscle. The muscles act as a protein reserve for amino acids, which provides fuel for the brain in times of scarcity. An equally important, but oftentimes overlooked, feature of muscle is its ability to remove glucose from the blood and store it as glycogen. Why is this important? If you recall, advanced glycation end-products (AGEs) are highly reactive and underlie many of the modern disease processes. Muscles act as a storage depot for carbohydrate and, in many ways, protect the rest of the body from the damaging effects of AGEs. For this system to function, however, one must:

1. Do enough physical activity to *build* some muscle.
2. Do enough physical activity to keep that muscle sensitive to insulin.

That second piece about insulin sensitivity is a bit of a lie—or at least a stretch. You see, when we exercise we turn on genes for a transport molecule called GLUT4 (remember that little bugger from chapter 3?). GLUT4 acts almost like a straw that spans the muscle membrane and allows glucose to be transported into the cell *without* the aid of insulin. Yes, even type 1 diabetics can make smart use of this alternate mechanism. What is becoming clear is that a significant portion of our blood glucose control should be handled by the GLUT4 mechanism. Normally we would be active enough to ensure that our optimal insulin sensitivity is maintained while also ramping up the GLUT4 pathway. This decreases the need for insulin, which decreases any of the collateral damage associated with elevated insulin levels. Remember, our hormones work best to promote health and wellness when they stay within certain parameters. GLUT4 helps to maintain optimum blood glucose levels while decreasing the need for insulin. And to activate GLUT4, we must exercise.

It should not come as a surprise that exercise benefits *all* hormones when the amount and type of exercise is correct. Let's look at a few of the better-known and more important of these hormones.

Growth hormone. Growth hormone (hGH) is critical for maintaining lean body mass, burning fat, and even fixing DNA damage. Its secretion is dramatically improved by brief intense exercise, low carbohydrate intake, punctuated eating (intermittent fasting), and restful sleep. HGH levels tend to decrease with age, but by emulating the exercise, food, and lifestyle of our HG ancestors, we can dramatically improve our production of the youth hormone.

IGF. Insulin-like growth factor, as its name implies, has activity similar to that of insulin, but the primary activity is anabolic, or growth, activity. IGF works synergistically with growth hormone to improve muscle mass and strength. IGF is also critical for the health and functioning of our most important muscle, the heart.

BDNF. For many years it was assumed that damaged brain cells do not repair, but the discovery of brain-derived neurotrophic factor and its effects on cerebral stem cells (cells that are similar to embryonic cells—they can literally become anything and respond to chemical signals such as BDNF) showed the brain is much more plastic and capable of growth and repair than we ever thought. Exercise is one of the most potent stimulants for BDNF production, particularly when coupled with smart nutrition and lifestyle.

This is a very short list of hormones beneficially affected by exercise. The point to take away is exercise is critical to maintaining normal hormone levels throughout life. The main difference between health and disease, vibrant youth or aged frailty, is one's hormonal profile. Your Paleo Solution will allow you to bring your profile into line with that of our remarkably healthy HG ancestors.

Now that we have looked at being strong and hormonally sound, let's take a look at your pump and pipes before looking at our exercise prescriptions.

Cardio!

It's almost impossible to talk about exercise and not have the topic shift to cardiovascular fitness. In fact, this is usually where the conversation starts and stops! For years it was assumed all we needed for health was "cardiovascular fitness." Those were the "running years," and health was emulated by a heart and lungs suspended in an emaciated bag of bones and scrawny muscles. So long as your heart was healthy, you were healthy—or so we thought. Thankfully, times have changed.

The Cooper Institute, which is the place that popularized the term *aerobics*, no longer recommends "aerobics" as it has been classically practiced. They now recommend strength training and interval training to provide not only cardiovascular fitness, but also an all-encompassing fitness, which includes strength, flexibility, muscle mass, and hormonal optimization. But I'm getting ahead of myself—let's look at the adaptations to the heart and vascular system that *are* of benefit, and then we will look at the best ways to get those adaptations.

Big Heart

Medicine can be a funny enterprise in what it regards as "normal." If you look at cardiac research, the "normal" heart is relatively small, particularly in the left ventricle (the main chamber of the heart to pump blood out to the body). This is the heart of a sedentary individual and for very odd reasons, this is considered the norm. If that same individual begins exercising consistently, the heart will change in response to those demands. The heart will enlarge, particularly the left ventricle. The wall of the heart will thicken, and blood vessels will grow in the heart muscle to allow better oxygen and nutrient transport to the heart muscle itself. This adaptation is called an "athletic" heart, and although it is recognized as healthy, it is not recognized as being the normal human heart. This is yet another example of genotype vs. phenotype. Our phenotype can be one of health (the athletic heart) or disease (the sedentary heart).

Nice Pipes

The heart is a pump that is attached to living, dynamic pipes. The arteries (carry blood away from the heart) and veins (return blood to the heart) respond to the activity of the heart, the nervous system, and hormones such as adrenaline. If you imagine the amount of blood in your body as being static, you can get a sense of how your heart and vasculature control blood pressure. If your arteries relax, the same amount of blood is now contained in a larger space, and this makes the blood pressure go down. If we constrict the arteries, it forces blood pressure up.

The net effect of exercise on the vascular system is it improves the ability to increase or decrease the volume of the vascular bed in response to activity. Most of you are familiar with a very popular drug, Viagra, which acts on the production of nitric oxide (NO). NO relaxes blood vessels. Exercise improves the cellular signaling which increases NO production, and this is part of the reason why exercise has benefits to sexual function similar to Viagra and related pharmaceuticals.

The net effect of exercise on the cardiovascular system is improved efficiency and "head room." An athletically enlarged heart is a more efficient heart. Each beat costs the heart and organism less energy, and requires less oxygen, as compared to a "normal" sedentary heart. This efficiency is further enhanced by improved vascular responsiveness. If you need to run to catch a bus, your heart, lungs, and vascular system work better and cost you less if you are fit than if you are sedentary. The "headroom" might also save your life. If you never exercise and you have an inefficient heart, you may not survive an unexpected bout of exercise or stress. If you are called upon to run for an airplane while hauling a suitcase and twenty pounds of extra you (that extra couple inches around the belly you have been ignoring), it's entirely possible to stress the heart to the point of failure.

Imagine two different cars towing a large trailer over a mountain pass. One is a four-cylinder, and the other is an eight-cylinder. Which engine typically has more horsepower to drag the trailer over the pass? Which car is more likely to fail due to lack of capacity? The human genetic norm is to have an "eight-cylinder heart." Lots of power, lots of capacity.

Bene<u>FIT</u>

So, from a big-picture perspective, exercise is literally woven into our DNA. We are born to be fit, strong, and healthy. We are supposed to look, feel, and perform like accomplished athletes. A significant proportion of our disease and early death is attributable to the discordance between our genetics and our sedentary existence.

As we dig into the details of our ancestral fitness, we find a balanced physique capable of most anything. Powerful muscles mixed with cardiovascular fitness was the norm for most of humanities existence. By emulating the amounts and types of activities of our Paleolithic ancestors, we can affect remarkable changes in our physique, mental outlook, hormonal state, and overall health.

Now that I have you whipped into an exercise frenzy, let's look at the different components of our Paleolithic Fitness. When you get to the exercise prescriptions, you will notice there are no machines recommended. You can certainly use machines if you like, but they offer inferior results with regard to balance, hormone response and, oddly enough, safety. Is *your* body the exact dimensions the machine is made for? If not, it is your joints and connective tissue that must accommodate the mismatch. Similarly, you will notice the movements I recommend are what exercise scientists call "compound" movements. We use these because they tend to mimic movements we see in sports and life, and they provide much greater return on our investment. If you are familiar with isolation movements and want to work them into your program, that is fine. Just focus on the full-body movements first, and then use your isolation movements as finishers.

Strength

Most people associate strength and "big muscles" with bodybuilders, football players, and chemists. OK, maybe chemists are not at the *top* of your list when you think about strength. But if you ask someone what "strength" is, they will usually relate strength (in the physical realm) to picking something up. From a physics or exercise science perspective, strength is the ability to exert force. Now, you may not have thought about it like this, but simply moving your fanny through the world necessitates a certain amount of strength. Have you ever seen someone who was quite frail who could not stand under his or her own strength? Someone who is that weak is very likely to have small muscles, poor blood sugar control, weak immunity, and, frankly, the person is at a high risk of sudden death. It is very likely the individual has little to no cardiovascular fitness because they simply cannot *do* anything.

People can debate what features of fitness are most important, but I'm going to put strength and mobility at the top of the list. If you have those two components, you can do just about anything. The nice thing about strength is it improves very quickly, even in the aged. Although there are different features of strength, which include adaptations by the nervous system, as well as changes in the muscle, we are going to focus mainly on strength improvements from a perspective of increasing muscle mass.

But, I'm a Girl!

If you are female and afraid of gaining muscle . . . oh, how to say this tactfully. Muscle, literally, is your friend. In the ten years I have been coaching men and women, *none* of the women grew into muscle-bound behemoths. Not one. If you recall the before and after photos and testimonials from the beginning of the book, women who work out and have muscle get lean and strong. They lose dress sizes and look great. As I've said before, some of this is nutrition, some is lifestyle, and some is working out—and that means gaining muscle.

I could cite endocrinology, epidemiology, sports science, and a number of other yawn-worthy topics in an attempt to convince you, but that is appealing to your rational intellect, and your fear of muscle is purely emotional. I'm stumped how to appeal to that other than this: if you have exactly the physique you want, do things your way. If not, strap in, quit worrying, and do it my way. My intention is for you to succeed, and part of that success is looking and feeling great. Oddly enough, it is not my intention to make you a contestant for a sideshow attraction. I have a feeling that would kill book sales! So please, like the food, just do what I recommend and then reevaluate. It *will* work if you give things a chance.

The development of strength is highly dependent upon how advanced a trainee is. Someone who is deconditioned will find they get stronger leg muscles simply from walking. Someone who has hiked, biked, and swam their whole life will need a stimulus like body-weight calisthenics or lifting weights to notice a strength increase. Someone who has lifted weights due to playing rugby or a similar strength sport for years may need very sophisticated programming to see improvements in their strength, as they may be reaching their genetic potential. So, strength is a relative thing. Everyone can improve it; almost no one has enough of it.

Power

From a training and athletics perspective, power is not just the ability to use strength, but rather the ability to use strength quickly. Picking up a 500-pound barbell in four seconds is a demonstration of fairly impressive strength. Picking up the barbell in less than a second is a stunning display of strength performed quickly: Power.

Sprinting, jumping, throwing, and changing direction while running are all demonstrations of power. It is worth noting, power is the physical attribute that deteriorates fastest with age. But it is also the fitness component that gives us the greatest rewards if we diligently train it throughout life.

All of us know people who are fast runners or exceptional jumpers. These folks tend to play basketball, football, or compete in track events under 400 meters. These people tend to have a high percentage of particularly explosive muscle fibers. We are all born with a variety of muscle fiber types, ranging from the slow but very fatigue-resistant type 1B fibers, to the very explosive type 2A fibers. Aging converts powerful 2A fibers to weak 1B fibers. You do not want this conversion from explosive to slow to happen. This change is synonymous with aging, which is why we will devote a significant amount of our time to developing not only strength, but also the ability to recruit strength blindingly fast. We want *power*.

It should not be surprising that many of the hormonal and cellular changes that occur with power training are also those of a youthful individual. We will see power development take a prominent role in intermediate and advanced trainees. Beginners tend to improve power by simply becoming stronger.

Flexibility (Range of Motion)

One of the most striking features of children at play is their flexibility. They seem capable of nearly super-human feats with no training or practice. Then we put them in chairs, and as time passes, their hamstrings and hip flexors shorten, eventually making a full squat challenging, if not impossible. Those children turn into us adults, but instead of realizing the error of our ways and getting out to run and play, we spend most of our time typing, reading, and writing from the seated position. Unfortunately these activities stoop us forward and tighten the postural muscles of the stomach, back, and shoulder girdle. The net result is a loss of the ability to move as children. This loss of flexibility, or range of movement (ROM) in medical terms, is made worse by poor diet and lifestyle (AGEs really stiffen up our otherwise pliable muscles and tendons) and undermines our strength.

Consider again the person who cannot easily stand from a seated position. Such people are not only weak, but also brittle. They look as if they might shatter if they fall, and oftentimes they do. Did you know that this degree of frailty and infirmity is virtually unknown in cultures where people sit on the ground for significant durations, such as in Japan? This is certainly a case of "use it or lose it," and yet another example of our modern world conspiring to age us prematurely.

We will improve your ROM in a holistic way, such that your joints and muscles are made stronger and safer because of your efforts. Flexibility work such as that practiced in many yoga forms not only can improve ROM, but also can dramatically decrease stress by entraining one's movement and breathing.

Endurance and Stamina

Endurance and stamina are used interchangeably, but we will make the same distinction exercise physiologists such as Dr. Jim Cawley make in this instance: *Stamina relates to local muscular work, while endurance is the ability of the heart and lungs to carry oxygen throughout the body.* Obviously these two concepts are kissing cousins, as you cannot stress the heart without doing work with the peripheral muscles, but when we look at our training, we will seek a balance in stimulus that *minimally* impacts strength, flexibility, and power. You see, cellular and neurological adaptations for endurance are antagonistic to those of strength and power—unless you structure your programming intelligently. We make smart use of interval training and circuit weight training to cause significant stress on the local muscular level. Using this technology we can maintain strength and power, while at the same time achieve remarkable levels of cardiovascular fitness.

Intervals

Let's do another thought experiment. Let's assume you have a large sum of money to invest, and you could invest it in one of two emerging technologies. Both technologies look pretty cool, but one of the companies can be proven to provide *eight times* the return on investment of the other company. Which one do you invest in? The decision seems obvious in this case, yet we have a similar scenario in the case of steady-state cardio vs. interval training, and people just do not seem to get it!

Hundreds of experiments have been performed comparing interval training (doing a certain amount of work such as running, biking, swimming, rowing, or jump-roping) vs. steady state training (doing the activity for a specific period of time). What is consistently found is intervals provide as good or better cardiovascular fitness as steady-state training, but with a fraction the time.

One study compared a protocol of twenty seconds of work, with ten seconds of rest, repeated eight times. Only four minutes of work total compared with thirty minutes of steady-state training. The interval group trained at levels that were harder than could be sustained (we call this type of training anaerobic), while the steady state group trained at 70 percent of the VO2 max (the VO2 max is how much oxygen one can use relative to his or her body mass). Any guesses on what happened? The interval group showed greater improvements in body composition (lost more fat) and greater improvements in both VO2 max and power production, and all with literally a fraction the training time.

Are intervals the only things you need to do to win a world championship in marathon or triathlon? No. You can use them to improve your training, and most smart coaches and athletes do just that, but if you want to be "elite," you need to do a significant amount of work at a steady state to become highly efficient at your chosen activity. If that is your shtick, fine, but do not fool yourself into thinking that tons of endurance training is going to optimize your health or longevity.

Do you remember my point that we tend to lose our fast-twitch muscles as we age? Endurance training *accelerates* this process. High-volume endurance work also depletes our body's store of antioxidants and subjects us to increased levels of oxidative stress.

Now, I'm just laying out facts here. Do not take this as a value judgment on your sport if you are into endurance athletics. I have a heavy bias toward the health and longevity side of things, so I bring that to my coaching and writing. Can a Paleo diet and smart training improve the performance of a high-level endurance athlete? Yes, absolutely. If you are interested in taking your endurance game to another level, I highly recommend *The Paleo Diet for Athletes* by Joe Friel and Prof. Loren Cordain. It is geared specifically for the endurance athlete, as are the numerous "Coaching Bible" books by Joe Friel. Joe is one of the most sought-after endurance coaches in the world, and he bases his nutritional approach on the Paleo diet.

Intervals sound pretty hard! Do I just jump in and go hard? Yes, if you want to kill yourself. Seriously though, intervals just mean doing some work and then resting. In the beginning, this may mean walking for one minute and resting for one minute. Over time, you may build up to running or biking, but as we will see in the Beginner Programming, the appropriate dose of exercise is very subjective. Take a small helping when you belly up to the "pain buffet."

Interval Weight Training Aka Circuit Training

Let's imagine yet another scenario: You are working in your backyard, loading thirty-five-pound bags of concrete into a wheelbarrow. Ten bags of cement go into your very burly wheelbarrow. Just as you finish the last bag, your dog sprints around the side of the house, obviously looking for a game of "Chase me, ya big dummy!" Being a big dummy, you chase your dog, corner him, and then turn and run, making your pooch chase you. Eventually, you get back to the wheelbarrow, grab the handles, and *lift!* You wheel the load around the side of the house to your front yard where you are working on a hideous bird-bath contraption the neighbors will hate even more than your life-size Battlestar Galactica statues you set up last year.

This whole process of loading the bags, chasing the dog, and toting the wheelbarrow took you perhaps ten minutes. If we had a heart-rate monitor on you to see what your ticker was doing during all this, what do you think it would show? Your heart rate and breathing would likely be very high at various points during these shenanigans.

Here is the funny disconnect, however: Although your heart and lungs are working very hard, most people do not consider this "cardio" and see little if any benefit in activities like this. This is an unfortunate loss, as exercise science has known since the 1940s that interval weight training (also called circuit training) is a remarkably effective means of building not only cardiovascular health, but also a significant degree of strength, muscle, and power.

We will make smart use of calisthenics, such as push-ups and sit-ups, combined with conventional movements found in the weight room, to build your Paleo fitness. We will also use some unconventional methods to keep you excited and challenged. Exercise might be hard, but it doesn't need to be boring!

Intervals Are Life

When we watch kids play, they naturally fall into intervals. Tag, hide and seek, and even most organized sports work in interval fashion. It is wholly unnatural for kids to just jump up and run 400 meters in one shot. Instead, they may end up running 4,000 meters while playing in the front yard over the course of an afternoon.

Animals tend to work the same way. A dog off-leash in a large park will run, scamper, sniff, and pee. Then scamper, run, pee, and sniff. Perhaps I need to start a fitness trend that involves frequent urination? Whatever the case, intervals, be they part of hiking or weight lifting, are literally part of nature. Can long, drudgerous hours build impressive levels of fitness? Yes, and it can make you so bored you quit or want to crash your bike into onrushing traffic. Fitness, like food, family, and friends, should be fun and support your life, not take from it.

OK, enough theory. Let's Work Out!

The Lifeline Program: A Little Goes a Long Way, and it Will Save Your Life.

It is impossible to write a general book that meets each person's exact needs according to where he or she might be. Some of you may be accomplished athletes, others have not broken a sweat in years. This book is largely geared toward the beginner—folks who might be sick, deconditioned, and not well acquainted with exercise or nutrition. The same principles do apply for the more advanced trainers and athletes. Restful sleep, a grain-free Paleo diet, and smart training are the keys to not only top level performance, but also optimizing health and longevity. For the sake of brevity, however, I will only provide recommendations on where to go next.

For the Lifeline program I am assuming that you have been sitting on your fanny a *long* time. I'm also assuming you are generally free of orthopedic issues, have a release from your doctor to begin a mild exercise program, *and* you have a little common sense. That means ramping up your activity slowly. If you are just lost, it might behoove you to get a knowledgeable trainer or strength coach to work with until you literally have your feet under you. The Lifeline program *seems* idiotproof, but people have "impressed" me at times in this regard, so use your good judgment!

I'm going to lay out several activities that you can do either singularly or in a circuit fashion, as well as many ways to alter the basic template for variety.

"Cardio"—Walking, Rowing, Biking, Swimming.

Hopefully these activities are familiar to you. Rowing might be new, but it is a highly effective training modality you might consider adding to the mix. Later, I'll give you some ideas on setting up a home gym, but do not get bogged down in the details here. If walking is the easiest and most accessible thing to do from this list, just stick with that. Folks get squirrelly and make squawking sounds about "boredom" in an attempt to avoid exercising, so I'll try to inject as much variety into this as I can. If you ride a bicycle, look both ways, wear a very flamboyant helmet, and try not to talk to strangers. Strangers scare me.

Lower Body—Squatting, Walking Lunges

There are quite a number of orthopedists, physical therapists, and other health professionals who will tell you squatting is "dangerous to the knee." If you ask these fine folks if it is dangerous to sit down, they will look at you like *you* are the idiot. Unless you are going on strike and never intend to stand up again, if you sit down, you will eventually stand back up. That friends, is called "a squat." Apparently, the medical profession would prefer you never practice *how* to squat and, instead, just pretend humans can navigate a life without squatting. It's madness and at the heart of the disconnect with our very nature. If your medical professional is very concerned that you are squatting, tell them you have switched to a much safer movement called a "sit-to-stand." In the mean time, let's look at how to squat, er . . . sit-to-stand.

SQUAT

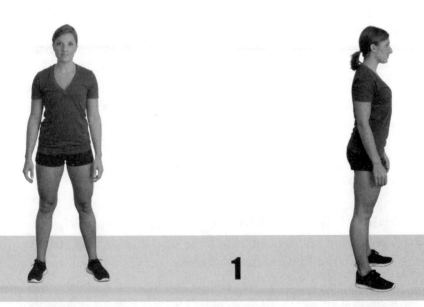

Stand upright with your heels under your shoulders, toes pointing slightly out. If you are new to all this stuff, place a chair, solid box, or similar object behind you. The object should be slightly higher than knee height in the beginning, just to be careful. We are simply going to sit onto that object, but with perfect form.

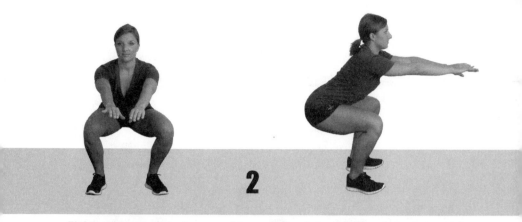

Tighten your stomach, fanny, and leg muscles. Get solid! Now, keep your weight in your heels, push your bottom back such that your knees track over your toes. Reach your hands forward for counterbalance. As your bottom reaches back, your knees track over your toes, and your upper body leans forward however much is necessary to stay balanced. Keep going down until your fanny contacts the chair, box, or whatever object you are using. Stop!

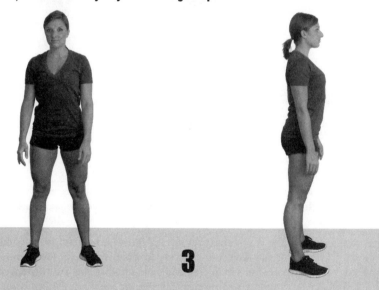

Now reverse the process, keeping weight in your heels, knees over your toes, and stand all the way tall with your hips back under your shoulders. You are now a graduate of the "Junior Squatter Club." Don't get too cocky, though; we have a little more work to do. Ideally, you are squatting with your hips just a little above parallel with perfect form. If that is the case, we will lower your box or chair progressively until you are performing a perfect, full-depth squat. Will this be hard for some of you? Yes. Flexibility and strength issues may make this a long process, but there is literally <u>nothing</u> you can do that is better for making you strong and healthy. Some people may need to use a very tall chair or box due to orthopedic or strength limitations. Use your best judgment and/or find a coach that knows what he or she is doing.

Walking Lunges

The walking lunge is most appropriate for someone who can squat full-depth for ten to twenty repetitions. If you are not at that level, save the walking lunge for later.

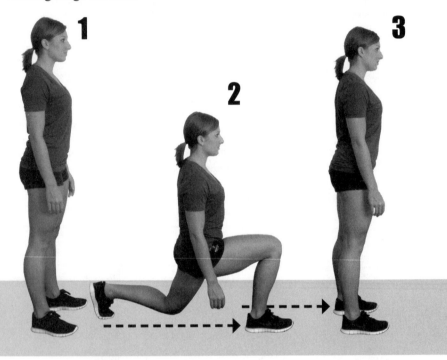

1) **To begin the movement, assume the same starting position as your squat. If you painted a clock on the ground in a circle around you, your nose would be pointing at "12."**

2) **Now step a leg forward. If you step your left leg forward, your left foot should land on the "11," and if you step your right leg forward, your right foot should land on the "1." The point here is to step wide enough that you are stable and balanced. This is not a sobriety test—unless, of course, you started this session with a few NorCal margaritas! You should step far enough forward that you can keep the shin of your front leg vertical (same as the squat, but avoid letting the knee go over the toe), but not so far that you have problems stepping the back leg forward.**

3) **Step your rear leg forward. You should alternate legs with each step. It is important to note that one leg may be much more stable than the other. Not to worry, that is why we are doing this! If this is a new movement, your "lunge" can be just an exaggerated step. Safety and progression are what count here. If you never knew quite where your gluteal muscles were, you will be able to draw a detailed anatomical diagram the day after you try these!**

Upper Body—Push-ups, Body Rows

You may not think you can do a push-up, but I'm willing to bet I can find a way to modify this classic callisthenic movement so that you can do it safely and effectively. If you are deconditioned or significantly overweight, we will start you from a standing position using a sturdy bench, counter, or even a handy wall. Let's start against a wall, which is the easiest way to do this, then progress to a more difficult version so you will understand how to scale this movement as you progress.

Wall Push-Up

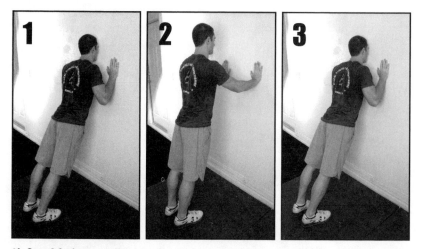

1) Stand facing a wall just a few inches away. Place your hands flat against the wall slightly below your shoulders, approximately at chest level. Now, step your feet back a few inches. Make your body tight from earlobe to toe-nails! Tighten your legs, bottom, and stomach.

2) Push yourself off the wall, fully extending your arms.

3) To return, allow your arms to bend, controlling your descent back to your start position. If you do this without paying attention, you will break your nose on the wall. I recommend against that. Now, try moving your feet back a few more inches and do a few more repetitions. Do you feel the slight increase in difficulty when you move your feet further back? This is how we can modify movements to make them safe and accessible to almost anyone. If this variation is easy, try using a counter or low bench or table, as demonstrated in the next sequence.

Chair Push-Up

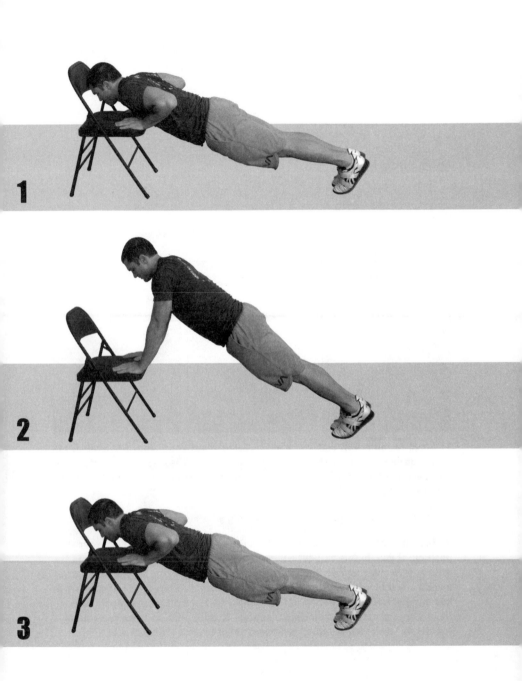

1) First make sure the chair is secure! Remember, you will lean your full weight against this object. If it moves, you might have a very short workout and a considerably longer rehab! Approach the chair the same way you did the wall. Feet are under your hips, your body should be tall and straight. Place your hands securely on the seat of the chair about shoulder width apart. Now, walk your feet back until the lower portion of your ribs is touching the seat.

2) Now, do a push-up! This should be significantly more challenging than the wall version but hopefully still doable for you. If not, you may need to spend your workout time mainly at the wall for now.

3) Slowly lower your torso back to the start position.

Hopefully the progression is obvious from here: By working your way to lower and lower objects you will be able increase your strength sufficiently to progress to a lower level. Eventually, you will be able to do a full push-up from the ground. It may take you week, a month, or a year—that will depend upon your situation—but you can make remarkable progress. The push-up not only works your arms, shoulders, and chest, but also the muscles of the back and stomach, as they stabilize your body during this movement.

Body Row

The body row can be looked at a few different ways: The opposite of the push-up or a modified pull-up. Whatever the case, the body row will become one of your favorite movements. Really! You will need to buy a little gear for the body row. A set of gymnastics rings, blast straps, or TRX system will all work just fine. You can find links for that gear and other items at the end of the chapter and on the Robbwolf.com website. You might have a local playground with rings that you can use for body rows, be creative!

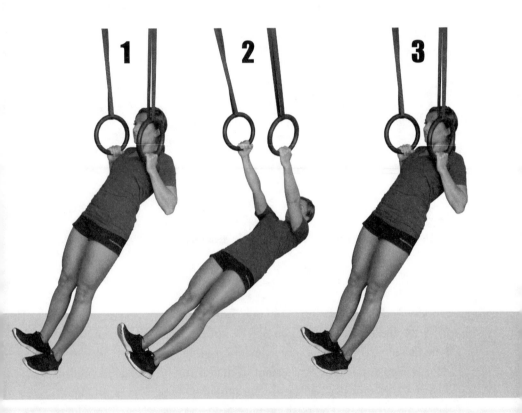

1) To perform the body row make sure your equipment is securely fastened to a mounting, as per manufacturer's instructions. Now, set the handles about armpit height. Make sure the handles are even in length so you do not end up with one massively developed arm. Grasp the handles firmly with your feet directly under the rings. Make your body rigid by tightening your legs, stomach, and back.

2) Now, slowly and with complete control, lower yourself backward. Maintain one safe speed throughout the movement, avoiding the tendency to "dive bomb" at the end of the movement. Your arms will come completely straight, keep your gaze between your hands to maintain neutral neck position.

3) Reverse the movement by squeezing your shoulder blades together while bending at the elbows, pulling your chest up to the rings. This should look much like a pull-up with the difference being your feet are on the ground and the movement is happening in front of you instead of overhead. Can you do a few repetitions at this position? If so, take a small step forward and see how this small change increases the difficulty of the movement.

Similar to the modifications with the push-up, the body row may be modified to meet almost anyone's needs. The final progression of this movement can be either a pull-up or a body row with your feet elevated on a box. We have used this same progression at NorCal Strength & Conditioning to help people in their sixties and seventies eventually attain their first pull-up *ever*. We have also used these movements in post operative rehab with people over 300 pounds. They are safe and effective if you tackle them with a bit of respect and common sense.

Get Dumb

Let's look at two very simple movements you can do with a set of light dumbbells (DBs) and then we will look at a beginners program.

Press

The DB press is simple and effective. You can perform this movement with a DB in each hand, or one hand at a time. To perform the press use a DB that seems too light in the beginning. It is best to establish flawless technique before progressing the weight.

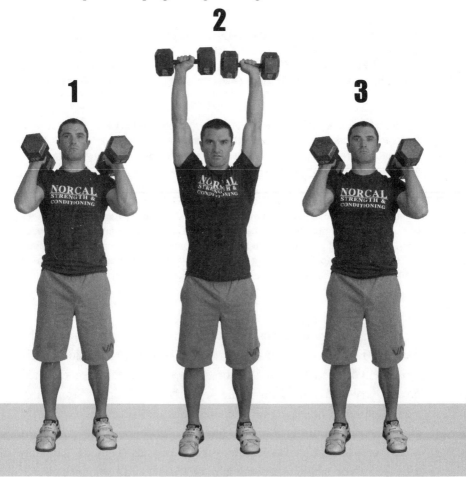

1) Lift the DBs to your shoulders, making sure you have a secure grip, your gaze is directly forward, and your elbows are directly under the DB. Your feet should be between hip and shoulder width, your legs, butt, stomach and back should be tight and steady.

2) Take a small breath in, hold it, and press the DBs overhead. Overhead should mean if we view you in profile, we can draw a line from the middle of the DB, down through your ears, shoulder, hip and ankle. The weight being held overhead should be held up like a column, straight up and down with no bending in any direction. At the top of the press your hands can rotate with the palms facing forward, forcing the heads of the DBs to lightly touch.

3) To return the DBs, allow gravity to pull the weights down, but use enough resistance to control the descent at a safe pace. The DBs will come to rest lightly on your shoulders with the palms facing each other (hammer grip again). Catch a few breaths and repeat. You should only hold your breath enough to stabilize your midsection, not enough to pass out! I suspect dropping a DB on your head or toe would really get your attention. Again, be safe and reasonable.

Dumbbell Row

You may have noticed a theme emerging, as we had two calisthenics movements (push-up and body row), a push followed by a pull. Similarly, we will strive for balance in our use of weights. You will use one DB at a time for this movement, and I recommend using your weak arm first (if you are right-handed that means use your left hand first).

1

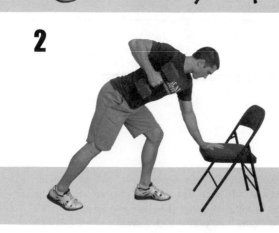

2

3

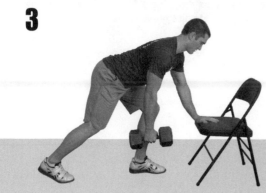

1) Let's assume you are left-handed and have the DB in your right hand. You will need to stand near a stable bench, table, or chair. You could simply use a wall but it is not quite as stable. With the DB in your right hand, take a fairly large step forward (similar to your lunge step you practiced earlier) and place your left hand on your chair or table. You should be leaning forward anywhere between your back being parallel to the floor to just slightly leaning forward. It is critical that your spine be straight and you do not hunch forward getting into, out of, or executing this movement. The DB should be hanging at your side with a tendency for the DB to rotate in.

2) Take a small breath in, brace your stomach, hips, and back, and row the DB up, initiating the movement by pulling your shoulder blade back. Simultaneous to this movement, begin bending the elbow and rotate the hand slightly outward. The "up" part of the movement is finished when you cannot raise the DB any further. Keep the back flat and facing the ground with your stomach and back tight and protecting your spine.

3) Lower the DB under control, taking a few easy breaths at the bottom of the movement when your right arm is extended. When you are ready to stand up you can set the DB down and stand up or walk the back foot forward, switch hands, and perform rows on the opposite arm. Remember! If you have the DB in your right hand, the left foot is forward and vice versa.

Program Modifications:
A Little Change Will Do You Good

Most people report that they do not exercise because of boredom. Physical discomfort and inconvenience are certainly factors, but the most common reason for abandoning a program is boredom. I hope the program laid out here will be fun and challenging, while taking up little of your time and avoiding boredom because of the variety. It may not provide much joy to know this, but when you are just starting out with exercise, *everything* works! Progress is quick and steady, the land of instant gratification. You just need to stick to it—don't do too much today, and do try to do just a little bit more tomorrow. Consistency, safety, and fun are the things to focus on. You will be amazed what a little consistency with your exercise will do when coupled with your nutrition and lifestyle changes.

I'm going to make a few assumptions here. They involve the notion that you have a certain amount of aptitude and competency with your movements. I'm assuming you know how to squat, lunge, body-row, push-up, DB press, and DB row. If you are comfortable with some of those movements, stick with those. If you are not comfortable with *any* of the movements, you are going to do a lot of walking!

Seriously though, you need to have a few different movements that you feel pretty confident in to change the basic program. I have worked with some very broken people who could walk, push up against a tall object (in our gym it's usually a gymnastics pommel-horse), and body-row. In the beginning our "warm-up" is simply doing a round or two of our chosen activity. If you have a kitchen timer or stop watch, that will help track progress.

Day One: Circuit Workout

Walk 200–400 meters. If you have no idea how far that is, walk one to two minutes out and then take the same amount of time walking back. Pick a landmark for this distance so you can track progress. Make it a brisk pace but within your means.

When you get back to your starting point, rest one minute. Then do five to ten perfect squats. (remember to use your chair or box for safety, if necessary). Rest one minute. Then do five to ten push-ups. Rest one minute. Do five to ten body rows. Rest one minute. Walk your same course again. You are done with day one.

How did you feel during the workout? Were you short of breath, dizzy, or very tired? If so, you might have gone a little too hard. The next day how do you feel? A little sore? Beat to heck? This will tell us how good your recovery is. We are shooting for a "little" sore. You know you did something because you can feel the muscles in your legs, arms, back, and chest, but you are not regretting your birth.

Day Two: Intervals

Walk, swim, or ride a bike. Shoot for ten to thirty minutes of continuous movement, but with the following twist: After you have warmed up at an easy pace for about five minutes, push your pace a little harder. It should be within your means, but sufficiently hard that you are looking forward to a break after ten to thirty seconds of work. After your first interval, ease back to a much slower pace. You may then cruise at this slower pace for thirty seconds to two minutes before kicking your pace up again. There is no perfect pace here; just push a little harder, then go a little easier. Try to keep moving forward.

If you are walking or riding a bike, you need to think about how far out you are going because you will need to turn around and come back! Remember, I am assuming you have done next to nothing for a very long time. If this is far too easy for you, jump to the Intermediate section. So, make a mental note of how far you went and how long it took you to cover that distance. You can keep a log of your efforts or simply write them on an index card taped to the refrigerator.

Day Three

Today is a bit of a rest day. Be active, but unstructured. Try to fit in some stretching. If you want to sign up for a yoga class or get a beginner yoga DVD, perfect. You are likely to be a bit tight and sore from your unaccustomed activities, but you should not feel "broken." If you do, you are pushing too hard and are likely to quit because feeling like you were pistol whipped gets old quickly. Ramp-up slowly and you will stick with it.

Day Four and Beyond: Circuit Day

This is a repeat of day one, but with the following change: If you felt "great" after your first day workout, shoot for ten reps on each exercise. If you are at that level already, do the same thing again, but take only fifty seconds between your exercises. Each time you do this workout, take ten seconds off your rest intervals until you have thirty seconds rest. When you reach that point, add a second *full* round. Walk, squat, push-up, and body-row. Each time you repeat the workout, decrease your rest by five seconds. When you reach fifteen seconds of rest and two full rounds, it's time to add a third round.

Now, each time you do this workout, decrease your rest by five seconds until you are doing three consecutive rounds. Once you can do three consecutive rounds, start making your squats, push-ups, and body rows harder. Get a lower box for the squats, until you are performing a full-depth, perfect squat in your workout. Push-ups will progress to lower boxes, eventually to your knees on the ground, and then full push-ups on the ground. Body rows will simply involve walking your feet forward. Once your body is at a forty-five-degree angle, you are doing about 50 percent of a real pull-up! This easy ramp-up will give you great results both in performance and in improving your body composition (you will look better naked).

If you were wrecked from day one, just repeat what you did and maintain the same rest intervals. Once you complete this workout without feeling like a punching bag, you can slowly step down your rest intervals. If ten seconds is too much of a step down, do it in five-second increments. Keep in mind, your feet need to stay in the same spot initially so you don't increase the loading prematurely. I want you to build your capacity at the easier positions, and then progress the loading.

Once you are down to thirty-second rest intervals, follow the progressions outlined above.

Day Five and Beyond: Intervals

This is similar to day two, but with the following twists: If you are already up to thirty minutes of activity, I want you to try to cover more distance in that same time. Remember, you are warming up by doing five minutes of easy activity and then stepping up the pace with intervals that are challenging but fun. I would like to see you cover more ground in less time for several weeks before we start kicking up the total time on this activity. I recommend this because people are usually time crunched. If you have a lenient schedule and feel strong on this activity, you can also add one or two minutes per session until you are doing forty-five to sixty minutes of continuous intervals. I am assuming you are still "walking" at this stage. If you are in fact walking, this means slower and faster walking (intervals). If you are biking, rowing, or swimming, think about your pace being described as slow or fast "walking." You will have a chance to sprint once you progress to the intermediate level.

If you started with ten to fifteen minutes of activity total, simply add one to two minutes of activity. Make a note of your increased distance so you can keep track of your progress. Each day you do this workout, add time until you are at thirty minutes. Then try to cover that distance faster. When you can shave two to five minutes off your time, start adding distance. In this way you can build up to forty-five to sixty minutes of continuous activity.

Day Six

This is your optional rest day. I recommend you do a little activity, such as some yoga or light stretching, but just go by feel. In a given week you will do at least one stretching/recovery day, but the second day is optional.

Day 7—Circuit
Day 8—Intervals
Day 9—Recovery

This basic template will serve you very well. You will improve your strength, endurance, mobility, and overall health. If you are following the Paleo Solution nutrition Rx, you should lose fat, gain muscle, and feel great. The combination of smart training and sound evolutionary eating will reverse insulin resistance and decrease inflammation. You will look and feel years younger while decreasing your likelihood of cancer, diabetes, neurodegenerative disease such as Parkinson's, and Alzheimer's, all while making your fanny look amazing!

With diligent work, this Lifeline program will allow you to reach pretty impressive fitness levels. You will be able to transition from walking to running at some point, and you will be capable of full push-ups from the ground and body rows that are almost parallel to the ground. At this point you effectively graduate from the Lifeline program to what my good friend, Dave Werner (who owns the outstanding gym, Level 4 Training, in Seattle, WA) would consider a "healthy beginner."

Now, you may have worked very hard to reach this point, and I fully applaud your hard work, but it's important to realize that you are just getting going. Remember how strong, fit, and capable our hunter-gatherer ancestors were? Remember how our genetics are wired for us to be just as athletic? The reality is this is a never-ending process, and we should all be a bit grateful for that. We have a lifetime of growth and opportunity ahead of us, and that should be pretty exciting.

It's important to be a little Zen about this process. Have a plan and a few goals that involve performance improvements, but keep your focus on today. Tackle the tasks and challenges at hand, keep it fun, and, *please*, don't make this drudgery! Many people feel overwhelmed in the beginning, but this is because they allow their minds to drift to the future. You cannot control the outcome—just your focus in this moment. Using the process of self-awareness and presence, you can accomplish amazing things, while also being happier in the only time you ever will really have: right now.

Keeping all that in mind, let's look at how to change your training before you fully enter the Healthy Beginner program.

Increase the Reps
It should be pretty obvious that you can begin adding push-ups and squats and body rows to your circuits. Progressing from three rounds

of walking plus ten squats, ten push-ups, ten body rows (thirty total for each movement) to three rounds of running plus fifty squats, fifty push-ups, fifty body rows (150 total for each movement!) is an impressive fete. It represents a simple progression that can keep most people challenged, literally for months or years.

Increase the Intensity

Let's assume you are competent at ten repetitions of your exercises in the three-rounds format. What if you just did one round, but as *fast* as you could? The intensity would increase dramatically, as would the hormonal response to the effort. For example, instead of walking, squatting, and doing push-ups and body rows with a break between each exercise, you perform them all back-to-back and then rest. The goal is to get adequate rest between every set so that you can tackle each effort with some chutzpah! This could be five minutes, or even longer. Keep in mind, this recommendation is for folks who are able to run, do full push-ups, and body rows and complete the three-round circuit. You can obviously increase the repetitions in this format as well, and this is actually a great way to get stronger at a particular element.

Ladders

A ladder is a slick way of packing a lot of training into a brief period of time. I was first exposed to this concept by Pavel Tsatsouline, author of the excellent book *Power to the People*. Let's use the squat, body row, and push-up for this example.

Here is how the ladder works: Do one squat, then one push-up, then one body-row. Then do two of each movement. Then three of each movement. Keep adding one repetition of each movement until you feel very challenged by a given set. Maybe you work up to six or seven repetitions in a round and you barely finish your push-ups or body rows. When this happens, simply start over at one. You could pick a set number of cycles to go through, like working your way up to five repetitions three times or do as many rounds as you can in ten minutes.

These are just hypothetical examples, but ladders usually take on this wavelike characteristic based on your motivation and fatigue. How hard should you push? Hard enough to feel challenged, but not so hard that you cannot move the next day. Ladders pack a lot of work in a brief period of time, so ease into them. You could use a day of ladders in place of your circuit-training days. You can also use alternate movements such as the walking lunge (a step with each leg counts as one rep), DB press, or DB bent row.

If you are particularly strong on one movement, you can keep it on its own schedule. Most people will be able to do far more squats than push-ups or body rows. You could easily keep your squats one ladder, working up as high as ten repetitions in a round, while your push-up/ body row efforts stay in the three-to-six range. This is all highly subjective, but it should provide a few ideas to get you going.

Wheel It!

This next activity will either make you popular or infamous with your neighbors! Get a sturdy wheelbarrow. Load a few rocks, cement bags, or other heavy items in it. Pick up the handles, and take a stroll. Children and small animals make pretty good ballast and have the added training stimulus of being an unstable ride due to the tendency for kids and critters to worm about. The downside, however, is that your ballast may simply jump out and run away. Use your best judgment here.

Although this type of activity does smack of yard work, it can be fun and remarkably challenging. Go for distance and see if you can get a little farther each time. When you are feeling sassy, add another rock or small child to increase the load.

I am often quizzed by my clients, "What muscles does this activity work?" My response is always to put them to the task, and then ask *them* what muscles are being worked. A good workout will make you an instant expert in applied anatomy, and pushing a wheelbarrow works most of the muscles from your earlobes to your toenails.

Bag It!

Get a backpack or weight vest and load it with ten to twenty pounds of weight. Walk out your door, preferably in a park or someplace with uneven ground, and just go. You can shoot for time or distance, but the main thing is to keep it fun and just move. If you are still significantly overweight, you may not need the additional weight. Yet again, use your best judgment here. An increase of ten to twenty pounds of body weight can make brisk walking as demanding as running. If you are ramping up and need a little more challenge, this is simple, fun, and effective.

It is important to note that you can substitute either of the above activities for your interval days. Keep it fun, but do keep some kind of progression in mind. Pick a distance and see how long it takes you to reach that mark. Try to go faster until you have cut 5–10 percent off your time. Then set a longer goal.

Bring a Friend

I'm going to share a sneaky way to ensure your success. Find someone to train with. I'd recommend a friend, coworker, or neighbor you get along well with. Family members can be . . . resistant. If you can rope a spouse or sibling into working out with you, good on ya, but a lot of people find family members to be tough to convince. Do not let your success hinge on the group of people in your life least likely to affect change. You will be able to find coaches, gyms, and online support at the Robbwolf.com website, but make a real effort to get a training buddy and keep each other accountable. You each need to state a few goals, be they performance oriented (I want to run a mile nonstop. I want to do twenty perfect push-ups) or aesthetics oriented (I want to fit into my favorite pair of jeans again). Goal setting, accountability, and community are critical to your success.

Get Dumber! The Healthy Beginner Program

As part of your Healthy Beginner program, I'd like you to start lifting more weights. The easiest, safest tool we can use for this is the lowly dumbbell. If you recall, the most important element to your fitness is strength, with a close second being flexibility/mobility. The DB is the perfect tool, as it allows us to perform a limitless number of movements using increasing loads and a full range of movement. Remember, start light, use good judgment, and focus on *perfect* form.

Squats and Lunges

Since you are familiar with these movements by this point, it should be easy to incorporate DBs into these outstanding lower-body movements. To load the squat, simply lift a pair of light DBs to your shoulders and perform your normal squat. Remember to stay "tight" by flexing the muscles of your stomach, back, and legs when performing the movement. Breathe at the top of the squat and brace your midsection while performing the movement.

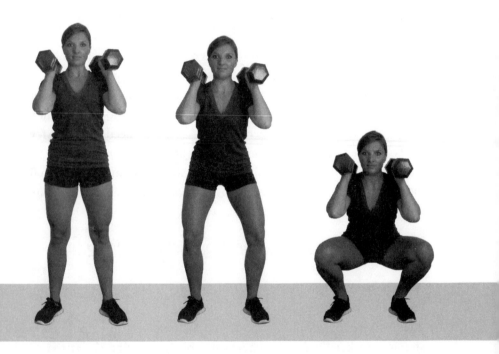

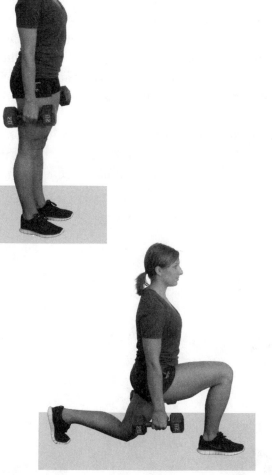

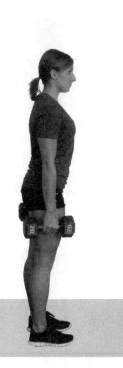

For the lunge, simply hold your DBs at your sides, keep your torso upright, and gaze straight ahead. All the cues from the basic lunge still apply: keep the knee tracking with the toe, make sure to step wide enough to maintain a stable base.

Bring Out Yer Dead!

One of the most basic of human movements, picking something up off the ground, has become a bit of a controversy in rehabilitation circles. Some claim the dead lift is dangerous and can hurt the back. Well, it *can*, but these same folks neglect to mention that the movement was once called the "health lift," and it was thought to be critical for long-term health and wellness. What has happened is people in rehabilitation and training have gotten lazy and a bit uncreative. Instead of teaching the proper use of this amazing athletic tool, we leave people—who might have been injured in the past working or doing other activities—to figure this stuff out on their own. Everything in life boils down to a risk/reward equation, and despite what the naysayers may claim, the dead lift offers far too much benefit to throw it on the scrap heap of training history.

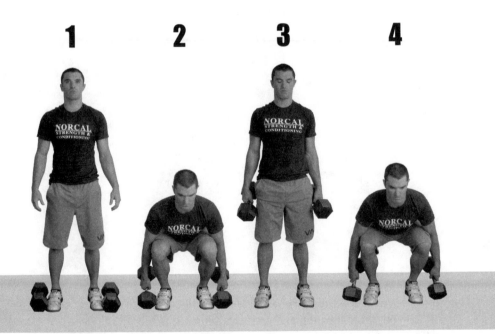

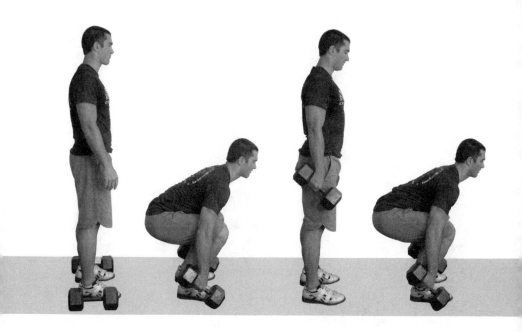

1) Here is how we will tackle the dead lift using DBs: If a pair of DBs are on the deck, approach them so that each DB is outside your feet and directly under your arms.

2) Take a little breath in, hold it, and bend forward, allowing your bottom to track backward and your knees to bend but not move forward. Unlike a squat, which tends to work the muscles of the frontal thighs, the dead lift, when properly performed, will work the muscles of your butt and hamstrings. If viewed from the side, your shoulders should be slightly in front of the DBs and your entire back is flat and strong.

3) You now push your weight through your heels, keeping the DB's close to your legs, perhaps even touching lightly. You will continue this movement until you are fully upright, with your gaze straight ahead.

4) To return the DBs to the deck, take a few breaths, hold a bit of air to stabilize your body, and push your bottom back, allowing your hips and the knees to bend but not track forward. If you have tight hamstrings or hips, you may find this movement challenging. If you do not have a perfect, full-depth squat, you may need to save the dead lift for another day. As I mentioned earlier, and as I will mention again, seeking a qualified coach or trainer can really simplify and accelerate the learning process.

Swing

The swing is a fantastic movement for developing the legs, butt, and midsection. If you perform a high number of reps in the movement, it can really get your attention due to its full-body nature.

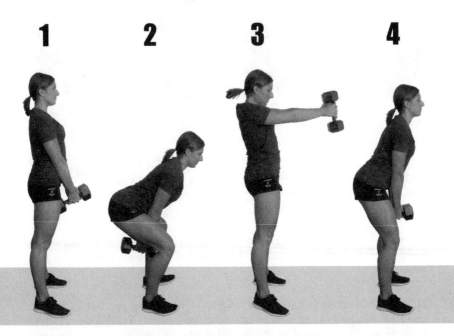

1) **Start with a very light DB, holding the handle in both hands as pictured. Depending on the size of the DB and your hands, you may find it easier to simply grab the top of the DB. Keep your torso erect, weight in your heels, feet about shoulder width.**

2) **Push your bottom back allowing the DB to swing back slightly.**

3) **Now, "jump" the hips forward, causing the DB to swing up to your navel or chest. The arms should merely guide the DB—they should <u>not</u> be the prime movers.**

4) **Do not interrupt its downward swing. Instead, allow your hips to swing back to "catch" the fall of the DB. This should involve very little movement on the part of both your hips and the DB. You should be able to store the energy of one swing and feed it into the next. Keep the amplitude (the size of your front and back swing) small until you are comfortable with the movement. If you perform the movement correctly, you should feel it in your butt and hamstrings, with no discomfort to the back.**

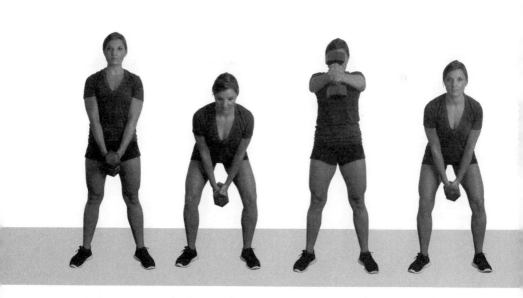

As you gain proficiency in the movement, you can push your bottom back a little more, allowing your torso to lean a little forward. This allows you to generate more power and, thus, propel the DB higher on subsequent swings.

Once you are comfortable swinging the DB to eyebrow height (you should be able to see in front of you when the DB reaches its max height), you can start adding weight to your swings. Progress slowly and carefully! Your first round of swings may make your next visit to the privy quite interesting! Sore hamstrings and bottom can make a trip to the toilet a "Zen-like experience"!

Push Press

The push press is a dynamic cousin of the press and one of my favorite movements.

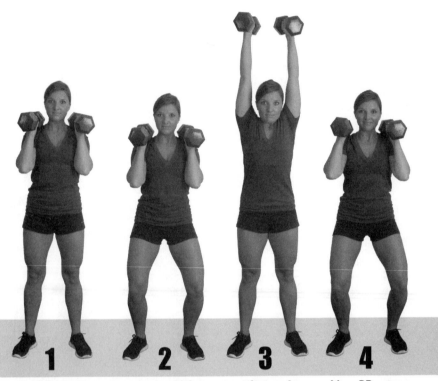

1) Start the same way you would for a press: feet under your hips, DBs at your shoulders, firm grip on the DBs, and your body braced for movement.

2) Now, bend your knees just a little, as if you were getting ready to jump. When you bend your knees, it is critical that you keep your torso completely upright and your gaze straight ahead.

3) Reverse the movement as if you were jumping and use the strength of your legs to drive the DBs off your shoulders and press them overhead. This is an explosive, but controlled, movement. Drive the DBs upward but slow them as you reach full extension of your shoulders and elbows overhead.

4) Pause a moment, and then lower the DBs under control. Once they are safely at your shoulders, you may bend the knees again and perform another push press. I actually breathe while moving if I perform the push press for high reps. Inhale on the down, exhale on the up. If your loading is sufficiently light, you will be able to do this as well, but if it is heavy or you are unsure of the movement, it is best to take a small breath in before you dip and hold the breath lightly until you return to your shoulders.

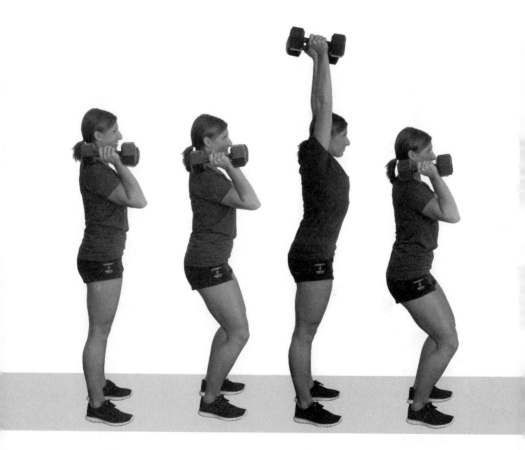

Ball Slams

This is a relatively inexpensive piece of gear that is actually fun. It's funny but most of our quiet, meek females expose their angry side when they start messing with the ball slam! The first few reps they still look dainty and demure, but by the fifth or sixth repetition the woman has transformed into some kind of killing machine savaging the poor ball! You may think I'm making this up, I'm not.

The ball slam is a full-body movement but you will mainly feel it in your butt and legs. It has a sneaky way of working your abs and shoulders also, but you will know that once you have played with it.

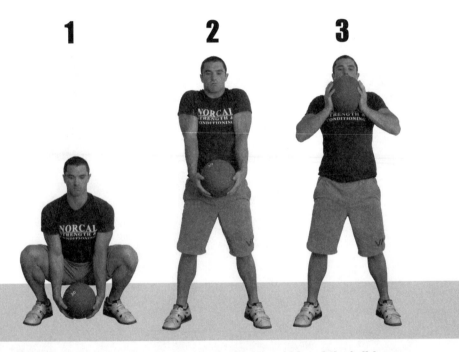

1 2 3

1) Approach the ball with your feet about shoulder width and the ball between your feet and about the middle of your instep. Reach down and grab the ball with your chin down, back flat, and weight in your heels.

2-4) Lift the ball by straightening the legs, pulling the ball into your body such that the ball rockets from floor to overhead in one smooth movement.

5-6) Now, keeping your weight in your heels, reverse the movement by tightening your whole body and slamming the ball back into the ground! Be ready, you need to follow the ball down and catch it on the bounce. Keep perfect alignment of your spine the whole way and let your hips "jump" the ball overhead and slam it down.

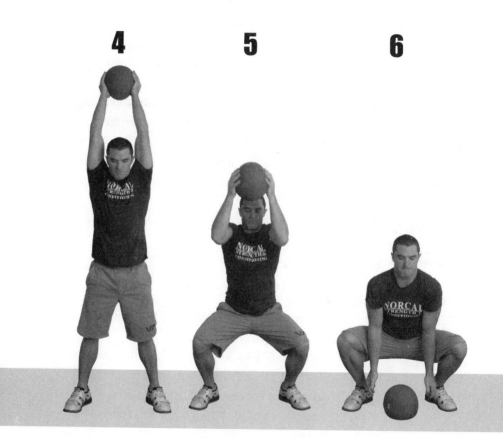

Important NOTE: Make sure you are using a ball like the kind recommended from the gear list. If you use a ball that has a lot of rebound, your first throw may be a trip to the hospital. The ball I'm recommending has little if any bounce. Be sure of what you are using, you will make this mistake only once!

Stepping Up the Healthy Beginner Program

Whether you are starting as what I consider a "healthy beginner" or you have battled to get to this place, it's time to step up your training. But how do you incorporate these new movements? Slowly and carefully. What I want you to do is pick one of the above new movements and practice it for five to ten minutes at the beginning of your workout. Practice ball slams, DB dead lifts, or a push press before you do your main workout. Now, when I say practice, that's what I mean! You need to pay attention to form, feel where your body is, and have your workout partner or partners critique your form while you critique theirs. Again, this is a great time to have a coach or trainer make sure you are on task here. For practice, do a few reps to see how the movement feels. Rest, make adjustments, and move forward. When you feel like you have mastery of a movement, start incorporating it into your training. When you have the DB dead lift mastered, switch it in for your air squat. When you have the push press, substitute it for the press or push-up.

Let's look at an example day to get you going.

Circuit Training

Let's say you are still playing with the ball slam but have "mastered" the push press and the DB deadlift. You might do a light jog for a warm-up and then throw the slam ball a few times, checking you position before lifting the ball off the ground, overhead, and upon release of the ball. Your training partner provides feedback and you do the same.

Now that the preliminaries are out of the way, it's time to have fun! You have a "200 meter" run that you have been using for your circuit days. It is actually a distance that you can run at a brisk pace in about one minute. You are doing this circuit with no breaks, just trying to complete the whole thing as quickly as you can, resting when necessary. You set your stop watch and you are off!

When you come in from your run, instead of squats, you begin with the DB dead lift. You are using a new rep scheme you thought of and do twenty DB dead lifts, then twenty body rows with your feet stepped forward such that your body is at a forty-five-degree angle with the ground. You need to break up the body rows. You do twelve, rest a moment, then six, rest a moment, and then finish the last two reps. You commit to yourself that the next time you do this workout, you will go something like twelve and eight reps! You then grab your DBs, get in perfect position, and perform all twenty DB push presses unbroken. You make a mental note that you will do the workout with DBs that are slightly heavier next time and then head back out on the run.

The 200 meter course you once had to walk, you are now able to run, even after the work you just did! You come in and do fifteen of each exercise, dead lift, body row, and push press, then head out for the run, and return and do ten of each exercise. After you finish your last repetition on push press, you push "stop" on your stopwatch. You note your time and how you performed the movements in your training journal. You also note the changes you want to make to your next efforts before doing a long cool-down walk and stretch.

Advanced Workouts

If you are a serious athlete who is oriented toward endurance athletics, I strongly recommend *The Paleo Diet for Athletes* by Joe Friel and Prof. Loren Cordain. I would also recommend Joe's other books in the *Training Bible* series. If you are a power-oriented athlete or simply a fitness enthusiast who is looking to optimize performance, health, and longevity, keep your eyes open for the forthcoming work *Fight Prep*, written by IFC Lightweight Champion Glen Cordoza and me. This book will provide advanced programming and nutritional strategies to maximize muscle gain, strength, and power.

In addition to this, I highly recommend you look at the following resources to expand your training:

* *Olympic Weightlifting: A Complete Guide for Athletes and Coaches* by Greg Everett
* Catalystathletics.com
* Coachrut.blogspot.com
* Movnat.com
* Gymnasticsbody.com

You can find additional resources at Robbwolf.com

Hey Robb

How should I eat to optimize my exercise results?

That is a fantastic question, but the answer is by necessity a little slippery. The reason why is pre- or post-workout fueling is fairly individualistic. Are you overweight? Lean and trying to gain muscle? A serious endurance athlete?

I'm assuming you are either a beginner and/or are getting back into shape, so fat loss and health are your primary concerns. Looking at the fueling question from this perspective, here is my "ideal" situation for you:

You work out in the AM before breakfast. If fat loss is your primary concern I'd make most of your meals protein, veggies, and fat (this may require that you modify the thirty-day meal plan that will be presented later in the book). Why do I make this recommendation? Because this approach will help you to lose fat and reverse inflammation remarkably quickly. Training on an empty stomach turns on some interesting genetic machinery that is important not only in fat loss but also longevity.

What if I feel shaky or lethargic during a workout?

Well, you may just need a little time to adapt, but you could have a little protein and fat (a small piece of chicken and a handful of nuts) before you train. This will work well, just not as well as the fasted training. Play with this and you will find an approach that works for you. As you become fit, your ability to train on empty will likely go up.

What if I cannot work out in the AM?

Obviously you need to work within the constraints of your schedule, but I find AM workouts to be particularly productive for fat loss. Just do the best you can, as it's more important to be consistent than stress over the details.

What if I'm a top-of-the-food-chain athlete who is lean and strong? How do I eat?

Again, this is somewhat specific to you and your goals, but you likely need more carbohydrate to support your high-intensity training. The best way to handle this is to make your post-workout meals protein and carbs. A few good examples of this include pork loin and sweet potato, salmon and blueberries, or London broil and water melon. Now you'd like to know how much protein and carbs to eat, yes? Two to six ounces of protein and twenty to seventy-five grams of carbohydrate brackets the needs of most athletes.

TEN

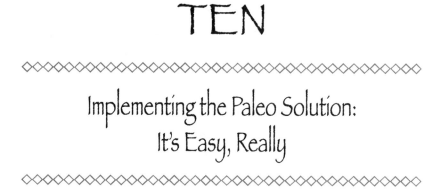

Implementing the Paleo Solution:
It's Easy, Really

I'm not sure how to introduce the following section, as it might contain the most important information you have ever heard. It might save or radically improve your life or the life of someone you know and care about. It is so damn simple, yet idiots and geniuses alike consistently miss the punch line. You see, the entire book up to this point could be considered a waste of time, as you really do not need to know *why* this stuff works to reap all the benefits. The information in this book, on my blog, and in the recommended reading is quite contrarian to the views of health and nutrition that are promoted by the government and media. I may make some money from this book, but even if it becomes a best seller, it's peanuts compared to the money to be made from pharmaceuticals. It's tough to patent an idea like: "Use the best that modern technology has to offer and then couple it with Paleo nutrition and lifestyle. Live long and prosper!" Lucky for Pfizer and Merck, their products are a lot easier to patent.

So, yes, this book has quite a lot of information to help answer the endless questions generated by this Paleo view of health, but it really boils down to the doing. In the ten years of helping folks with their nutrition and fitness, I have observed that people fall into one of the following categories:

1. About 50 percent of the folks I work with "get" how to eat Paleo immediately. The Paleo concepts make sense, they modify their cooking seamlessly, and they never look back. They live a Paretto kind of life in which they adhere to things about 80 percent and actually get about 95 percent of the benefit Paleo has to offer. Folks with serious health problems (myself included) follow a tighter plan because they find the increased diligence to be worth the results in how they look, feel, and perform. This is a simple ROI (return on investment) analysis, and a little common sense and the observational abilities of slime mold can tell you where on this spectrum you need to be (fully compliant, or a dabbler). God bless this 50 percent because I really earn my money on the other 50 percent!

2. About 25 percent of folks fall in the DUMBB category (Dude, yoU Must Be Balanced!). These folks argue every damn point of minutia and claim that we need to be "balanced." Should we ignore the fact that these "experts in balance" have no exact definition of what "balance" means, or any explanation of why they are still sick and overweight? They have enough excuses to win a congressional filibuster. But at the end of the day, it's all fluff. Eventually I wear these people down and get them to simply try things for a month. They tend to battle and find ways to slow the process. (Shouldn't I have a bound food log? Or maybe an online food log to document my meal? Or maybe if I wear pink leotards it will make my ass look smaller and I won't *need* a food log.) These folks need some hand-holding in the kitchen, supermarket, work, school, and social functions. And we need to keep them accountable, lest they wander off and become vegan or something goofy like that. But they eventually stick with the program and see significant results and success. When this happens, these folks become OMGWTH-STHUAP (Oh my God will they shut the Hell-up about Paleo!) As hard as it was to get them on board, they are so ecstatic about their success, they become annoying even to my trainers and me. Just the cost of success I guess!

3. The final 25% (I'll keep their acronym to myself—it's *not* very nice) battle the process the whole way. They have baggage that is apparently more fun than success and progress. It's Mommy issues, Daddy issues, self-esteem issues. It's a fear of change, and it all plays out the same way. They want attention, they do not comply, they fail to make progress. I want to lobotomize myself with a pencil. I try to help these people, but I'm no therapist, and I don't want to be. I understand many of the mechanisms on a social, biochemical, and even an evolutionary level, but at some point, you've got to realize that you can't save everyone. If you insist on being helpless, your needs will exceed my abilities to help you, and I will move on to the other 75 percent who want to succeed. The only difference between this group and the previous group is these people will not even try this for a month. They are a month away from transforming their lives and from success, but they just won't do it.

All We Are Saying . . . Is Give Paleo a Chance

So, I want to make this as easy as possible. I want it to work for you and your goals. To this end, I've laid out a tiered plan that will allow you a level of buy-in that works for you. But I'm *really* going to hard sell, as if your life depends on it. Just for a month. I want you to understand how powerful this Paleo concept can be in our life. Do you have a serious autoimmune condition, cardiovascular disease, or depression? Well, you need tight compliance guidelines *if* you want to be healthy. Always been lean and strong and generally can eat anything and still remain pretty healthy? Cool, I hate you (just kidding!), but you *will* benefit from a Paleo approach to eating. You will likely have a bit more latitude with your eating and lifestyle than someone who is sick, but you will still reap significant benefits.

The reason I recommend tight compliance for about thirty days (for everyone) is because this will give your body an opportunity to fully adjust to the foods it was meant to run on. It will give you a chance to assess how you look, feel, and perform. My website has grown in traffic and our gym has grown in members for one reason, and it's not because I'm a snappy dresser or a witty conversationalist. OK, I do have the gift of gab, but the reason for this growth and success is simple:

Paleo Works

It works better than anything else. But you need to give it a chance. In this vein I frequently get the question, "Does Paleo work for X?" With X being one of the following: Fat, skinny, old, young, pregnant, athletic, nonathletic, sick, healthy . . . you get the idea. My response?

Paleo works, but only if you *do* it.

Let's tackle this implementation thing in a graded fashion so we can keep you out of that final 25 percent! Now, I'm not only going to show you *how* to do this, as in what to eat, how to cook, how to shop, but I'm also going to give you solid biomarkers you can track so you and your doctor know this stuff is working. If what I'm proposing is solid, you should not only look, feel, and perform better, we should be able to track biomarkers of health and see them go in a favorable direction. Easy, right?

Go Forth and Shop!

I love our clients. Really. I tell many funny stories about our motley crew, many of which poke fun, but without them, our gym would just be weights, gymnastics rings, and crickets. Even though I *love* our clients, I am occasionally flabbergasted by some of the self-defeating strategies they cook up to make their lives difficult. Sometimes it gets so bad, I consider if I want to go on living at all! Case in Point: One of our top trainers has been working with a woman, I'll call her Lysa, for about three months. Lysa has been fun like a root canal in a Third World country while dealing with a bad case of jock-itch. Lysa had an excuse for everything and, ultimately, ended up in the final, unreachable 25 percent. Interestingly, Lysa's extreme obstinacy and unwillingness to change has inadvertently helped thousands of people. You see, one day, in an effort to make small talk, I asked Lysa, "How ya doing?" to which she replied, "I don't know how to shop *this* way. I don't know how to cook *this* way. Lysa strongly emphasized "this." In fact, it came out more like "thiiiiiiiiiiiissssss." If you could cross the word "this" with the sound made by fingernails on a chalkboard, that would be pretty close.

Autoimmune Caveat

If you know you have an autoimmune disease or if you have a significant amount of pain and inflammation, I recommend you take your Paleo Solution to a higher level. Don't run away, this will just be for a month or two, so we can see if some common foods might be problematic for you. Now, I'm not talking about grains, legumes, and dairy. We already discussed those, and if you have health problems, I hope you understand those foods are not your pals. What I'm talking about are some otherwise "Paleo" foods that can pose a problem for some people. These foods include:

- Eggs
- Nuts and seeds
- Tomatoes
- Potatoes
- Eggplants
- Peppers

So why are these foods a problem? In addition to the foods we have already talked about, the foods I've listed here have similar potential to irritate and damage the intestines of some people. So, if you have autoimmune or inflammatory issues, remove these foods and see how you look, feel, and perform. A remarkable number of people who have taken this extra step have reversed or significantly improved their inflammatory issues.

Oh, man, I was had. "Just walk away, Robb, don't ask!" I thought to myself. But I am a sucker for this stuff and went for it.

"Lysa, what do you mean you don't know how to shop *this* way?" To which she replied, "You know . . . *THIIIIISSSSS Thiiiiisss Paaaaaaleeeeo Stuff!*" Same nails on a chalkboard, combined with the following movements: Imagine locking your arms at your sides, except at the elbows. From the elbows down you can move. Now make your arms spin around at the elbows by kinda flopping your head and hips back and forth, somewhat like a convulsion. Think about a street mime choking on a martini olive. Equal parts "the show must go on" and universal sign for choking.

I approach coaching as a small bit of performance art, and I was *not* going to be outdone in my own gym! I asked Lysa, "Have you *ever* bought eggs or bacon?"

"Yeeeessss," Lysa responded, arms still spinning.

"Lysa, have you ever bought fruit and veggies? Salad fixings or stuff to grill?"

"Yesssssss."

"Lysa, have you ever bought a steak, seafood, ribs, or pork loin?"

"Yeeessss."

"Well, Lysa, you damn well do know how to shop like thiiiiiisssss."

Our clients love me, ask them. I think we have about six.

The point to this? It would never have occurred to me that someone would try to pull the "I don't know how to shop *this* way" card. What Lysa did was inspire me to write a shopping and food guide. You can find that here: Robbwolf.com

You need to download this, print it out, and take it with you. If this is too much trouble, take the damn book with you. That way, when you go shopping for meat, seafood, veggies, and fruit, you know what meat, seafood, veggies, and fruit means! No excuses, Buttercup!

So, you have downloaded the shopping and food guide from Robb-wolf.com and you are heading out to do some *serious* foraging! You can tackle this like a game or a military campaign—that's up to you. But for the most part, you will confine yourself to the perimeter of the store. Imagine that the interior of the store is packed with bean-burrito-eating vegetarians. Beans, vegetarians . . . don't make me get graphic here! The interior of the store is your foe, unless you are buying detergent, coffee, or cat litter.

Produce

Your first stop is the produce section. You will focus more on veggies than fruit, especially if your goal is significant fat loss. Athletes and folks who are already lean can get away with more fruit and starchy tubers like yams and sweet potatoes. More on that later.

Buy what is in season. Watermelons are *not* in season in North America in January! If you have a local farmers market, hit that and you are all but assured of buying local and in-season produce. Organic? Fine, go for it, but do not use a lack of organics *or* a prohibitive price on organics to forgo fruits and vegetables in favor of brown rice or Little Debby Snack Cakes.

This is one of the common arguments from the DUMBB camp: "I can't find organic lettuce, so I'll just get a sandwich and pasta." Oftentimes people strive to be perfect just so they can "fail" and give up. Don't do it—don't complicate this stuff. Tackle the refinements in steps so you do not get overwhelmed. Work to get color from the entire rainbow: Red, orange, yellow, green, blue, purple. You need not have that color spectrum represented at every meal, or even in a given day, but in a week you should see variety from all these colors and the produce they represent.

Benefits

There are no essential carbohydrates. Push your dietician or doctor on this topic, and then watch him or her squirm as the truth emerges. Then see the qualifiers come pouring out! Although carbohydrates, unlike fats and proteins, are not *essential* to life (we can make our own, thank you), they can be highly beneficial. Fruits and vegetables have an amazing amount of nutrition to offer above and beyond their relative carbohydrate content. In addition to vitamins, minerals, and antioxidants, they contain a host of novel substances known to fight cancer, diabetes, and symptoms of aging. If you were to compare a 1,000 calories of fruits and veggies with a 1,000 calories of supposedly healthy whole grains, you would find that grains do not provide the RDA for much of anything, yet fruits and vegetables look like taking a nutritional supplement. We've done this analysis for you, and you find it at Robbwolf.com.

Flavor of the Day

Make sure to include things that fall more into the flavoring category like ginger, basil, cilantro, onions, shallots, garlic, peppers, mint, and rosemary. There are a ton of other herbs, spices, and similar items that are available fresh, so stock up. Be adventurous! You will need these later in the kitchen.

What About Fiber?
Won't I Forget How to Poop Without Grains?

Fiber? If I had a nickel for every time I was asked where we get fiber in the Paleo diet! How about fruits and vegetables folks? Look at the fiber content in the comparison in Table 3 on page 219. Our dieticians would have us believe fiber comes only from bran muffins and brown rice. Do you see how dumb this is?

Meat and Seafood

Your next stop should be the seafood section. There are a few considerations when buying seafood, as there are mercury bioaccumulation issues with larger species such as tuna and sword fish. Look to fish like sardines, mackerel, and pacific salmon—smaller, shorter-lived fish tend to accumulate far fewer toxins. Shellfish such as shrimp, mussels, and clams are excellent and wildly underutilized. Many species of fish such as petrale sole are barely known in most of North America and Europe, but they are amazingly tasty and represent sustainable fish stocks unlike other, slow to reproduce varieties.

Go Wild!

Look for "wild" when you are buying fish. You may pay a little more, but quality matters with fish: High omega-3 to omega-6 fat ratios makes wild seafood anti-inflammatory as compared to farmed fish that are fed refined grain products. Similar to organic produce, the wild-caught issue should not be a deal breaker, but if you have a choice, wild is the superior option.

Meat/Poultry

The meat section is easy: find leaner cuts of conventional meats (which tend to be cheaper) and stock up! London broil, pork loin, lean ground beef, whole or parts of chicken (breast and thighs), turkey (same as chicken). People get into trouble when they fail to plan ahead and are

Eggs: How Many?

Eggs . . . hmmmm. I don't know what the deal is. Maybe it is be-cause these ossified orbs come from the hindquarters of chickens, but they sure do stir up a lot of controversy. First the medical es-tablishment tells us the cholesterol content is more dangerous than Russian roulette with a Howitzer, then we hear we should just limit them to less than six per week. And as I said above, eating eggs when you have an autoimmune condition is not recommend. So what is the deal? Will eggs kill me? I don't see a need for an upper or lower number in regard to egg consumption. I highly recommend omega-3-enriched eggs, and I also recommend that they not make up every single breakfast that you eat from now until the end of time. They can be problematic from a food allergy standpoint, but their benefits and convenience far outweigh any hazards.

left with no easy options at home. Round things out with some omega-eggs.

Free-Range/Organic/Grass-Fed

This topic gets a little dicey, so drink some espresso and hang on! "grass-fed" might mean "organic." Organic, as a standalone label claim, almost never means grass-fed. Free-range may or may not mean much of anything. Here is how this really breaks down:

Grass-fed

This typically refers to beef, bison, and similar grazing animals. It *should* mean that all the critter has eaten is grass and similar nongrain feed. Why does this matter? Because grains make critters fat and sick (just like us). It alters the omega-3/omega-6 fat ratios. Too many ome-ga 6s can make us inflamed. Grain-feeding animals irritates their di-gestive system, which creates a Mengele-esque race against time: The animals get so sick from eating grains, it's a race to get them fat enough for slaughter before they *die* from digestive complications. Not only is this a huge drag on resources (it is wickedly inefficient to raise corn to feed to cattle), from an ethics perspective, it's pretty damn disgusting.

My wife and I were recently vacationing in Nicaragua, and *all* of the meat was grass-fed and absolutely amazing in quality. Why was it grass-fed? Because Nicaragua does not have a government that subsidizes both agriculture and oil in a way that makes it economically viable to feed its herds corn. Yet I'm sure we will export this nasty habit as we are slowly eroding the grass-fed meat industries of New Zealand and Australia.

Most vegetarians give up meat because of the way animals are treated. Opting for grass-fed meat is perhaps the largest step you can take to make an economic vote for how your food is produced. Grass-fed animals require virtually no antibiotics and are far healthier than their grain-fed counterparts. Most of you may not know this, but the occasional outbreaks of dangerous E. coli bacteria are caused by grain feeding and sloppy slaughter practices. Normally, E. coli is relatively benign, and it is easily killed by our stomach acid if we are unfortunate enough to ingest it. Grain feeding, however, gives cattle acid reflux, just like us. This high acid environment selects for varieties of E. coli that are acid resistant. This means the E. coli is *not* killed if we eat contaminated food. Add to this the sloppy slaughter practices common in most large-scale commercial facilities, and you have a nasty, dangerous situation that could be solved by grass feeding and hygienic slaughter practices. You can change all of this by voting with your food purchases.

Organic

Organic is a somewhat nebulous term that describes production methods, usually involving nonsynthetic pesticides and fertilizers. Organic is a nice concept, but for me it lacks a pragmatic perspective. Some of the "natural" pesticides are more toxic than synthetics. Plutonium is "natural," but it is not good for you! People get a little Earth-motherly on this topic and fail to use some solid science from toxicology and other disciplines to make smart, informed decisions.

All that said, organic is a good concept overall, but you need to keep your wits about you when buying meat. Organic meat has likely just been fed "organic" grains. Same problems of n-3/n-6 fat content and other issues, but with a remarkably higher price tag. Organic and grass-fed are not typically government subsidized, so you pay more for them. Do you want to pay top dollar for meat that has the same goofed-up n-6 fat ratio as standard meat? Didn't think so. When we start talking pork and poultry, things get murky. You need to do a little investigating as to the feed of a particular variety. We have a local pork producer who feeds the critters almonds, oranges, and apples. It makes for amazing pork quality, but this is not a widely available product . . . yet!

On Robbwolf.com, you will find a list of CSAs and resources to buy grass-fed and organic products. Much of this process is predicated on education. If you ask for grass-fed meat, someone will provide it.

Why All This Meat, Seafood, and Poultry?

Well, because that's what you are designed to eat. Your physiology runs best on a high-protein intake. Protein from animal sources provides the basic building blocks for your muscles, plus many of your hormones and neurotransmitters. Meat and seafood is also incredibly nutrient dense: B-vitamins, zinc, iron. Calorie for calorie, lean, grass-fed meat is tough to beat.

Hormonally, animal protein releases glucagon, which not only helps to regulate energy levels, but also helps to maintain insulin sensitivity. Barry Sears, Author of *The Zone* and several dozen spin-off books, makes the claim that protein balances insulin release because of the glucagon release. This is, well, wrong. Foods are additive. Carbs release quite a bit of insulin; protein can range from a little to a lot, depending upon the source. But the combo most assuredly does *not* reduce total insulin released from a meal. The insulin response from a meal is an additive affair and protein + carb + fat = a larger overall insulin response, not a smaller one. This is why we recommend most meals are protein, veggies, and good fats, as low glycemic load veggies release relatively little insulin. For now, just keep in mind that dense protein sources are nutritious and beneficial for their satiating and hormonal balancing effects.

But What about Beans and Rice? What about Vegetarians?!

Hey, who let you in here? Oh well, what's done is done. This question always comes up, might as well answer it. Most vegetarians will dismiss the need for meat as one can combine foods such as beans and rice or corn and squash and construct "complete" proteins. If only that worked. You see, most plant-derived protein sources have an incomplete profile of amino acids. Humans have eight essential amino acids (amino acids we must get from the diet as we cannot make them) that are plentiful in animal sources and lacking to various degrees in plant sources. Many agricultural societies found that certain combinations (like beans and rice) can prevent protein malnutrition. Kinda. Remember the Hardin villagers? They, like most vegetarian societies, are less healthy than hunter-gatherers and pastoralists. This is a fact. Plant sources of protein, even when combined to provide all the essential amino acids, are far too heavy in carbohydrate, irritate the gut, and steal vitamins and minerals from the body via anti-nutrients. Remember that whole chapter on the double-edged nature of grains and legumes? Beans and rice, nuts and seeds, are what I call "Third World

Butter

So, what's the story with butter? It's dairy, right? Therefore on the Paleo "no fly" list? Well, butter is dairy; it can present some problems for folks with autoimmunity because of the milk protein content and lectins that are still a part of the butter. Sorry hippies, even clarified butter (ghee) is a problem. I would, however, put grass-fed butter on the "occasional" list. The fatty acid profile is better (lower in palmitic acid, much higher in CLA) and the antioxidant content is nothing short of impressive. Butter is mainly fat, so if we clean up the lectin problem, and push the fatty acid profile toward that of healthful grass-fed varieties, it's tough to build much of a case against grass-fed butter unless you have autoimmunity. See, I'm not a zealot after all.

proteins." They will keep you alive, they will not allow you to thrive. Your protein needs to have the following criteria:

1. It needs a face.
2. It needs a soul.
3. You need to kill it, and bring its essence into your being.
4. Really.

But You Did Not Address Vegetarians!

Oy vey! Ok, I'll address some of the ethical and environmental fallacies later in the book, but if you insist on tackling this vegetarian style, here is how you do it: Try to make things look as close to Paleo as you can. Use *dense* protein sources like these: tofu, tempeh, brown rice protein, pea protein. No TVP, no seitan. Why? They are loaded with gluten! Add lots of good fats and loads of fruits and veggies. Add to this a final ingredient:

Prayer.

Not to get all spiritual or New-Agey, but you might want to call on any gods who might be kind to your cause. You will not lean out, perform, or gain muscle on a vegetarian interpretation of Paleo when compared to an animal protein–based approach. I've seen hundreds of people try; it does not work as well. It is a good bit better than a high-carb vegetarian diet, but folks still tend to have autoimmune, GI, and inflammatory problems on the vegetarian approach.

Think I'm full of hooey? Fine, do it my way for a month, monitor how you look, feel, and perform, track your blood work, then do it your way. I did not make the rules to this game, I'm just informing you as to what they are. So get in and either prove or disprove things for yourself.

Your cart should now be brimming over with produce, meat, seafood, and poultry. You are almost ready to split this scene, but you need a few more items! This *will* involve a foray into the guts of the store (stay *out* of the cookie aisle). While you are there, you can grab a few bars of 85 percent dark chocolate, some red wine, and a good bottle of Tequila. A caveman/woman needs to party, right? Oh, yeah, double back to the produce section for some limes. Lots of limes.

But the real reason for being in the center of the store is this:

Oils and Spices

Olive oil: Two varieties are smart here. Get an inexpensive variety that you can use for cooking and a pricey variety that you use raw to top salads or meals that have been plated and are ready to be eaten. Olive oil quality varies widely and the regulations on what can be sold as "extra-virgin" are a joke. You need to do some label reading and educate yourself if you want to get your money's worth. I highly recommend Pacific Sun (http://www.pacificsunoliveoil.com/) for your high-end variety. It is made by a small family farm in Northern California, and the quality is second to none. Remember, olive oil is a great source of monounsaturated fats and disease-fighting phenolics and antioxidants.

Coconut oil: Coconut oil is a short-chain saturated fat that is delicious and perfect for higher-temperature cooking. If you cannot find a good variety locally, you can order it from tropicaltraditions.com

Coconut milk: You can find this in the Asian foods section of most stores or take a drive to an Asian food market. Coconut milk is delicious in curries and stews. Coconut has potent antimicrobial action and helps to heal irritation in the digestive tract. But mainly, it's delicious.

Herbs and spices: In addition to the fresh herbs you grabbed in the produce section, you need to stock up on some of the dry stuff. The shopping and food guide has an extensive list, but shoot for fifteen to twenty herbs and spices. Why so many options? Because many people like to play helpless and complain. I'm not going to let you undermine your success, and variety is important for long-term compliance. Go pay for all this stuff and then I'll meet you in the kitchen. It's time to get cooking!

OK, So What Do I Fracking Eat?

Like I mentioned earlier, owning a gym and working with people for years has been fun, rewarding, and at times damn confusing. Folks come to you with a problem—let's say they want to lose body fat and get lean. We start working with the person, introduce smart exercise, and begin educating them on what they need to eat to succeed. We talk about sleep and stress. These people *seem* to get it. And then they get home and have no idea what they are doing. We give them shopping guides. We give them recipes. But somehow the excuses and ability to be helpless wins out.

Do you remember Lysa? Lysa not only did not know how to shop, Lysa was also somehow *bored* with eating Paleo even though she hadn't really done it since she didn't know how to shop. You can only imagine how *that* conversation went. So, something I tackle with all my clients, and something we will look at with y'all right at the beginning, is what I call the Food Matrix. In addition to providing you with the thirty-day meal plan, I am also going to help empower you. You know the old saying about teaching people to fish vs. giving them a fish? Well, Buttercup, you will soon be a master at preparing Paleo meals.

Here is how this works: We have a list of fifteen meats, fifteen veggies, five fats, and twenty herbs and spices. These are all easily available from your local grocery store. It is perhaps unreasonable to have *all* of this on hand in your home, but it is reasonable to have at least five different protein sources and five different veggies. Now, the cooking oils and the herbs and spices—there is no reason not to have at least that much variety in your home. It is, folks, unconscionable to have fewer than twenty herbs and spices in your cupboard. Punishable by public caning.

OK, back to our example. If you take one item from each of these columns and consider that a meal, you have 22,500 meal options. If that was one meal a day, you would potentially not see the same meal for *sixty-one years*. So much for boredom! Most of these meals will be damn good, and it is nearly idiotproof easy: Put some oil in a pan, start browning meat, add herb or spice, then add a vegetable. Cook for five to ten minutes. Eat. Granted, there will be a few dogs in that list. The salmon-lard-Brussels sprouts-cinnamon combo sounds absolutely horrid. But hey, you will not see it again for sixty-one years!

Do you see how much variety there is here? It's staggering. And we are only talking about taking one thing from each column. What if we allowed for combinations? Then we are talking about literally limitless variety from this small list of ingredients.

So, the Food Matrix is both helpful in a very real sense—you can construct real meals using this simple tool, but it is also an antidote. It will literally save you from your own BS. You are not bored, you are lazy. You need to buy some pots and pans, some protein, veggies, herbs, and oils, and get your fanny in the kitchen and cook.

Say that again . . . I cannot understand the mumbling.

You are saying you do not have time? How about our contributor, Sarah Fragoso, who has three kids, two dogs, and a husband who owns a screaming busy chiropractic practice? She works and just finished her BS in psychology. Sarah cooks. She uses the Food Matrix, pots, pans, slow cookers, and pressure cookers. Sarah did not succumb to the BS, and she and her family reap the benefits at every meal. Of course, she does not have much time for TV, video games, or other wasted endeavors. If you want this, you find ways to do this. Check out Sarah's kitchen wizardry at www.everydaypaleo.com.

Time Crunched

I know, I know. Everyone gets busy. Here is a great resource for you to get Paleo-friendly snacks (grass-fed, gluten-free jerky), as well as prepackaged, frozen meals delivered to your door. The menu only includes dishes that are built from grass-fed meat, wild-caught fish, and organic vegetables.

www.paleobrands.com

Robb, You Are a Big Meanie!
I Have No Idea Where to Start!

So, perhaps you have literally never cooked before. You literally cannot even peel a banana. If the meal is not out of a box or stuck between two slices of bread, you have no idea what to do. Well, you are really going to make me work for this, aren't you? OK, let's make this easy and start with breakfast. Breakfast tends to be a tough meal for many people anyway, so let's start there. I learned of this technique from a well-known strength coach named Charles Poliquin. He starts his clients with a "meat and nuts" breakfast. Now, this can literally be "meat and nuts" (a piece of London broil and a handful of almonds) or this can be scrambled eggs and avocado or some chicken-apple sausages and some coconut flakes. It is a solid, sustaining breakfast that sets your hormones and neurotransmitters for the day. Add to this a triple espresso, and you are ready to get some serious world saving accomplished!

Do the meat and nuts breakfast for a week. Then tackle your lunch. Make the lunch look like breakfast, but add some vegetables. Make it a salad of grilled, steamed, or raw veggies. Run with breakfast and lunch for a week. Then add dinner. Make dinner look like lunch. There you are, Buttercup! You are all grown up and eating like a big-Paleo kid!

Now, this graduated buy-in is absolutely critical for some people. They just can't get their minds around the "whole Paleo thing" in the beginning. So we will tackle it in steps. Obviously, you can get straight to the goods and just make all your meals Paleo. If you are sick, overweight, or autoimmune, I'd highly recommend that, but again, that's all up to you. I will, however, go through a little exercise like I did with Lysa, and I'll ask you a few questions:

Q: Have you ever eaten some eggs and bacon for breakfast?
A: Yes.
Q: Have you ever eaten a salad with some chicken or grilled fish for lunch?
A: Yes.

Q: Have you ever had some meat or seafood with veggies for dinner?

A: Yes.

Well, kiddo, you have, on separate days, already eaten several weeks, if not months, of "Paleo meals." You simply have not strung them together to the exclusion of crap food. You *do* know how to do this. You *can* do this. It's simply a question of *will* you do it.

Fruity?

Notice that I did not mention fruit. Most folks are battling some kind of metabolic derangement, aka obesity, diabetes, fertility issues, depression, etc. This with a mixed bag of autoimmunity and systemic inflammation. Until you are lean and healthy, you don't get much fruit. There is no nutrient in fruit that is not available in veggies, and fruit may have too many carbs for you. When we start talking about what constitutes "health," we will see where on that spectrum you are. For now, just keep things simple and you will reap the greatest rewards.

One final thing needs to happen to ensure your success—and it's so important it should come *before* you go shopping. You need to get your affairs in order.

Clean Out Your House

Even though the vegetarians decry meat as a health scourge, no one, I mean *no one*, lies in bed at night thinking about the pork loin in the refrigerator. They do think about the ice cream, cake, or cookies. My friend, Kelly Starrett, has a saying: "Best self-defense: Don't be there." This is particularly true when we are talking about food.

You see, you have *no* self-control when it comes to food. Some may do better than others, but the reality is our ancestors never faced the types of foods we pack into our pantries. The sugar, the refined carbs. They are completely new and they are addictive. We worked with a woman who was, no joke, addicted to crack at one time. She overcame that addiction only to succumb to a massive sugar addiction. She started working on her food, and in her own words, she found kicking sugar and refined grains to be much harder than quitting crack.

This may sound preposterous, but the same receptor sites in our brains that respond to heroine and opium (the opiate receptors) are triggered by wheat. This combo is made more powerful when there is sugar present. Junk food is *really* addictive. You need to plan if you want to succeed.

Many of you will start on this path, but you will leave some junk in the pantry because "the kids will have a fit without it" or your spouse will similarly "lose it." Guess what? They do not need it either, and if you leave it in the house, it will suck you in and you will not make the progress you otherwise could.

Remember, I'm recommending that you give this a full try for thirty days. If vibrant health and a lean strong body are not what you want, you can always go back to what you were doing, But what I'm trying to do is ensure that you succeed. You do not get to blame your failure on your family.

You may want to dismiss this stuff, but think about it like this: Most people feel like they can stay in a monogamous, lifelong relationship. Sure, giving up the dating life might cut a little excitement from your Saturday nights, but there are other benefits to a long-term relationship. Well, what if we dropped you off at the Playboy mansion (I don't care what gender or sexual orientation you are), and let's say we got you falling down drunk and dosed you to the gills on Ecstasy. Would you remain monogamous? Highly unlikely, and this is my point: refined carbs are like an ecstasy-soaked beer binge at the playboy mansion. This is a battle you will not win, so stack the cards in your favor. Bag up all your crap food, take it to your local shelter and, I guess inadvertently, contribute to the death of the homeless. Well, better them than you.

But Raaawwwwbb, How Will I Get My Vitamins? And How Will I Poop without My Fiber?

Nutrient comparisons:

Let's check out some interesting information generated by my mentor, Prof. Loren Cordain. What I want to look at is the fallacy that grains, legumes, and dairy are nutritious or that you will be missing something if you do not have them in your diet. Most people have been brain-washed into believing the only place we can obtain vitamins, minerals, or fiber is from the government-sponsored grain-a-thon. So, let's look at these common misconceptions and counterpoints to help put this all in perspective.

Misconception 1:
Grains and dairy are particularly nutritious.

Misconception 2:
One will experience some kind of deficiency without grains, legumes, and dairy in the diet.

Misconception 3:
The only place to get dietary fiber is grains and legumes.

And this last point is not so much a misconception as a serious lack of understanding on the part of dieticians: One should eat a low-calorie diet. Now, I'm not arguing about the calorie content per se, but rather how they tackle it, as you will see.

Let's look at the following tables and do a little thinking. Table 1 comes from: *Origins and evolution of the western diet: Health implications for the 21st century.* Am J Clin Nutr 2005;81:341-54.

In the far left-hand column we have a list of vitamins and minerals. In the other columns you will find various food categories and how those foods rank for specific nutrients (this is comparing equal, 100-calorie portions). The ranking system is on a scale from 1 to 7, with 1 being lowest and 7 being highest. What we observe is that whole grains and milk are not particularly nutritious on a calorie-per-calorie basis as compared to meats, sea foods, veggies, and fruits. This one chart handily addresses misconception 1 (grains and dairy are nutritious) and it implies that if we are considering nutrition on a calorie-by-calorie basis, grains and dairy are not the winners. What if we look at this data represented as a modern interpretation of a Paleo diet? Luckily, Prof. Cordain has both asked and answered this question (see: L Cordain. *The nutritional characteristics of a contemporary diet based upon Paleolithic food groups.* J Am Nutraceut Assoc 2002;5:15-24).

TABLE 1

Mean nutrient density of various food groups (418-kJ samples)[1]

	Whole Grains	Whole Milk	Fruit	Vegetables	Seafood	Lean Meats	Nuts and Seeds
Vitamin B-12 (µg)	0.00 [4]	0.58 [5]	0.00 [4]	0.00 [4]	7.42 [7]	0.63 [6]	0.00 [4]
Vitamin B-3 (mg)	1.12 [4]	0.14 [1]	0.89 [3]	2.73 [5]	3.19 [6]	4.73 [7]	0.35 [2]
Phosphorus (mg)	90 [3]	152 [5]	33 [1]	157 [6]	219 [7]	151 [4]	80 [2]
Riboflavin (mg)	0.05 [2]	0.26 [6]	0.09 [3]	0.33 [7]	0.09 [4]	0.14 [5]	0.04 [1]
Thiamine (mg)	0.12 [5]	0.06 [1]	0.11 [3]	0.26 [7]	0.08 [2]	0.18 [6]	0.12 [4]
Folate (µg)	10.3 [4]	8.1 [2]	25.0 [6]	208.3 [7]	10.8 [3]	3.8 [1]	11.0 [5]
Vitamin C (mg)	1.53 [3]	74.2 [5]	221.3 [7]	93.6 [6]	1.9 [4]	0.1 [1]	0.4 [2]
Iron (mg)	0.90 [4]	0.08 [1]	0.69 [2]	2.59 [7]	2.07 [6]	1.10 [5]	0.86 [3]
Vitamin B-6 (mg)	0.09 [3]	0.07 [1]	0.20 [5]	0.42 [7]	0.19 [4]	0.32 [6]	0.08 [2]
Vitamin A (RE)	2 [2]	50 [5]	94 [6]	687 [7]	32 [4]	1 [1]	2 [3]
Magnesium (mg)	32.6 [4]	21.9 [2]	24.6 [3]	54.5 [7]	36.1 [6]	18.0 [1]	35.8 [5]
Calcium (mg)	7.6 [2]	194.3 [7]	43.0 [4]	116.8 [6]	43.1 [5]	6.1 [1]	17.5 [3]
Zinc (mg)	0.67 [4]	0.62 [3]	0.25 [1]	1.04 [5]	7.6 [7]	1.9 [6]	0.6 [2]
Sum rank score	44	44	48	81	65	50	38

1 Food types within food groups are based on the most commonly consumed foods in the US diet (135, 136). Values in brackets represent relative ranking (7=highest; 1=lowest). The micronutrient concentrations for each food group were derived from reference 64. RE, retinol equivalents.

TABLE 2

Sample 1-day menu for a modern diet based upon Paleolithic food groups for females (25 yrs, 2200 kcal daily energy intake).

	Food Quantity (g)	Energy (kcal)
Breakfast	-	-
Cantaloupe	276	97
Atlantic salmon (broiled)	333	605
Lunch	-	-
Vegetable salad with walnuts	-	-
Shredded Romaine lettuce	68	10
Sliced carrot	61	26
Sliced cucumber	78	10
Quartered tomatoes	246	52
Lemon juice dressing	31	8
Walnuts	11	70
Broiled lean pork loin	86	205
Dinner	-	-
Vegetable avocado/almond salad	-	-
Shredded mixed greens	112	16
Tomato	123	26
Avocado	85	150
Slivered almonds	45	260
Sliced red onion	29	11
Lemon juice dressing	31	8
Steamed broccoli	468	131
Lean beef sirloin tip roast	235	400
Dessert (Strawberries)	130	39
Snacks	-	-
Orange	66	30
Carrot sticks	81	35
Celery sticks	90	14

Let's next consider table 2, which lays out a sample 2,200-calorie meal plan composed of lean meats, seafood, fruits, veggies, nuts, and seeds. If you notice, there are no processed foods in this plan—but is it nutritious? Will you keel over and die from a plan like this? Is your doctor's or dietician's fear accurate that you will develop horrific deficiencies on this plan? Will your bum forget how to poop without "whole grains" providing fiber?

What we notice in table 3 is pretty interesting: 42 grams of fiber from these wacky things called "fruits and vegetables." Also interesting is the fact that our essential fatty acid ratio (n-3:n-6) is 1:1.5. In other words, "perfect."

TABLE 3

Macronutrient and other dietary characteristics in contemporary diet based on Paleolithic food groups for females (25 yrs, 2200 kcal daily energy intake).

Protein (g)	217
Protein (% energy)	38
Carbohydrate (g)	129
Carbohydrate (% energy)	23
Total sugars (g)	76.5
Fiber (g)	42.5
Fat (g)	100.3
Fat (% total energy)	39.0
Saturated fat (g)	18.0
Saturated fat (% total energy)	7.0
Monounsaturated fat (g)	44.3
Polyunsaturated fat (g)	26.7
Omega 3 fat (g)	9.6
Omega 6 fat (g)	14.2
Cholesterol (mg)	461
Sodium (mg)	726
Potassium (mg)	9062

The really interesting information is in table 4. If you notice we not only meet the recommended daily allowance (RDA) of all the vitamins and minerals (with the exception of calcium, which I'll discuss in a moment), but we have anywhere from several hundred to a thousand times the RDA. It is well understood that the RDA is a minimum and likely does not reflect an optimum nutrient level for performance, health, and longevity. Interestingly, however, we do not see significant health improvements from nutritional supplements (more on this in the supplement chapter). Epidemiology consistently shows consumption of nutrient-dense foods to be beneficial, not vitamin pills.

Now, as to the calcium issue, this is simple chemistry. Look at how much magnesium we obtain on this plan. Calcium and magnesium work synergistically in the body, and if our magnesium intake is high, our calcium needs dramatically decrease (see supplement chapter for further details).

TABLE 4

Trace nutrients in a modern diet based on Paleolithic food groups for females (25 yrs, 2200 kcal daily energy intake).

	TOTAL	% RDA
Vitamin A (RE)	6386	798
Vitamin B1 (mg)	3.4	309
Vitamin B2 (mg)	4.2	355
Vitamin B3 (mg)	60	428
Vitamin B6 (mg)	6.7	515
Folate (μg)	891	223
Vitamin B12 (μg)	17.6	733
Vitamin C (mg)	748	1247
Vitamin E (IU)	19.5	244
Calcium (mg)	691	69
Phosphorus (mg)	2546	364
Magnesium (mg)	643	207
Iron (mg)	24.3	162
Zinc (mg)	27.4	228

ELEVEN

Tracking Your Progress

There are two possible outcomes: if the result confirms the hypothesis, then you've made a measurement. If the result is contrary to the hypothesis, then you've made a discovery.
—Enrico Fermi

Blood is not thicker than money.
—Groucho Marx

We have come a long way together, but we are not finished yet. And not to be mean, but this is *your* fault. How so? Here is what I've observed working with people: They will give the Paleo Solution a shot, look, feel, and perform better than they have in years, and then talk to a know-it-all friend, family member, or doctor and get scared that a lack of grain will somehow kill them. So, we need to take some measurements and offer up proof, whether it is to pacify your curiosity or quiet your physician who has yet to connect the dots between evolution, biology, and medicine.

So, what types of things might we measure and why? Well, we will start with simple measurements like photos and a few dimensions that we can take with a standard measuring tape. As they say, photos do not lie, and the information we gain from a simple waist/hip measurement can tell us more than thousands of dollars of diagnostic blood work. Speaking of blood work, we *will* look at key markers of health and disease and educate you on how to ask for tests your doctor may not know about. I'll help you interpret these tests, as well as tell you what to do if your numbers are not looking so great.

Keep in mind that any nutrition and lifestyle approach that is worth doing should *not* have "side effects." If what we are doing is sound, we should look, feel, and perform better. We should be able to track biomarkers of health and disease (blood work), and we should see this go in a favorable direction. Easy enough, right? Well, let's look at the easy stuff, then move to the blood work and biomarkers.

Photos

This process is so simple it hardly seems worth mentioning, but a remarkable number of folks who begin an exercise or nutritional program fail to adequately document or quantify progress. Photos should be taken in the same clothing. Ideally, clothes that are formfitting, light in color, and show some skin! This outfit does not need to be something that you feel comfortable sharing on Facebook—it's something you will use to evaluate *your* progress. Take the photos from the same position and make sure you document a front, side, and back photo. A close-up of your face in profile and straight on is also helpful, as we tend to lose fat from our face and neck first.

You can update these photos weekly, and then make them into a slide show to really get a sense of your progress. Remember! Consistency is critical for the photos to really help you judge progress. Changing your placement, clothing, or lighting will alter your perception of the change. If you are too embarrassed to get help with the photos, use a mirror to take them—just keep the camera out of the way! Remember, this process is for you! You can share the photos if you want, or hide them in your secret place. That's up to you. Just to recap:

1. Take photos in the same clothing. Make the clothing formfitting where appropriate. Nonexistent clothing is even better.
2. Get front, side, and back photos.
3. Get a close-up of your face, both frontal and profile.
4. Update photos weekly and make sure to label them with the date if your camera does not automatically do this.

5. Stand in the same place when taking the photos.

Tape It

It may be surprising, but a simple measuring tape may offer more insight into your metabolic health than an extensive battery of blood work. The waist-to-hip ratio (WHR) is the measure of the narrowest portion of the waist (typically at or slightly above the belly button) divided by the widest portion of the hips. In general, the hips of both men and women will be greater in diameter than their waist. As you might have guessed, there are ancestral norms here that we can use to give us some guidance. Measurements of .9 for men and .7 of women seem to correlate well with health and wellness, to say nothing of attractiveness. So, what happens to our numbers if the waist gets larger and what might cause that?

Well, if the waist gets larger, it makes that number approach 1 (or even more than 1 in certain situations), and insulin resistance is what causes this increase. It should not come as a surprise that a waist-to-hip ratio that is too large is associated with everything from periodontal disease to cancer and heart attack. It is a simple, visible measure of insulin-resistant fat. So here are the steps to figuring out your own waist to hip ratio:

1. Measure your waist at the narrowest point. Use your belly button as a reference point and thread the tape around you, meeting again at the front. You might find it easiest to use centimeters. I'm still embarrassed that the United States is using inches, but it will not matter so long as you are consistent with either inches or centimeters. Now, repeat that measurement three times. Each measurement should be pretty darn close, but we will use a little statistics to keep us honest. After you have your three measurements, add them together and divide by three. This will minimize any errors you have in your measurements and it will earn you a "Jr. Scientist First-Class Award." This is your waist measurement.

2. Measure your hips at the widest part. Repeat the measurements three times, add the measurements together, divide by three. Just like for your waist. This is your hip measurement.

3. There is a rule in publishing that you will cut your readership by 50 percent for every equation you have in a book. Well, here goes: Take your waist measurement and divide it by your hip measurement.

4. High-five your bad self. You have now calculated your waist–to–hip ratio.

5. Track this number every two weeks. Try to take the measurements at the same time of day to minimize variables such as fluid retention. Women may see some variability in WHR due to changes in their menstrual cycle, but this variability will decrease with dietary and lifestyle compliance, as excessive water retention will cease to be a problem when ancestral norms in insulin levels are maintained.

What Does It All Mean?

A WHR of .8 and above for women and .95 and above for men would indicate an increased risk of diseases related to insulin resistance. Cancer, diabetes, heart attack—remember the insulin chapter? In my opinion, perhaps the most important measurement you can take is simply your waist circumference. Decreased waist circumference? Good. Increased? Bad. Pretty damn easy, and this works not just for dietary compliance, but any type of insulin resistance, whether caused by poor food choices or elevated cortisol due to excessive exercise or inadequate sleep.

Blood Work

I see this section being relevant for several types of people or situations:

1. It provides guidelines for those of you who are geeked-out on your health. You want to do everything "right," and this will provide the tight guidelines you desire.

2. To help bring your doctor on board. I beat up on doctors a fair amount in this book, but the reality is most doctors legitimately, sincerely want to see their patients get healthier. *But* they also get their primary education after medical school from drug companies. Doctors are not used to patients who take an active role in their health, so when you suggest an "unproven" dietary and lifestyle approach, they get nervous. The blood work should help because we can predict what should happen when you change your nutrition and lifestyle and then confirm these changes via time-tested lab values.

3. This section is also good for those of you who still think meat and fat will kill you. Many of you are coming from a vegetarian camp. All I suggest is you follow the recommendations in this book for a month, and compare your blood work before and after doing this. Easy enough, right?

Most of the blood work we need comes with a standard blood test. There are a few add-ons I will suggest to help paint as accurate a picture of your metabolic health as we can. One could easily spend thousands of dollars on diagnostic blood work, but to what end? If you look, feel, and perform better; if we bring a few of your biomarkers into ancestral norms; if we can show a marked decrease in your systemic inflammation by adopting a few simple nutrition and lifestyle changes, then why complicate things? It's your money, so spend it how you want to, but I'd rather see a vacation than blood work. I'm just silly that way.

Order Up!

You will need to work with your doctor to get this blood work ordered. You need to make absolutely sure that your blood work is performed in a *fasted state*. All doctors should know this, all testing labs should know this, but I cannot tell you how many people have spent money on blood work that was useless as the samples were taken in a nonfasted state. Shoot for at least a nine- to twelve-hour fast. Let's look at what to order and what those tests mean.

The Basics: This stuff comes with most blood work.

Total cholesterol
HDL
LDL
Triglycerides
Glucose

Add-ons:

LDL particle size
Glycated hemoglobin (Hba1c or just A1C)
C-reactive protein

Total Cholesterol
What Is That?

This is a measure of several blood lipid fractions that are in part proteins used to shuttle fats and cholesterol around the body. For simplicity, they are lumped under the general term "cholesterol." This includes
VLDLs (very low-density lipoproteins), LDLs (low-density lipoproteins), and HDLs (high-density lipoproteins). As we will see, each of
these categories of lipoproteins has specific physiological roles, as well
as their own subcategories.

How Much?

We are looking for numbers between 120–140mg/dl on cholesterol.
This reflects our ancestral norms, the range we see in all primates, and,
interestingly, all newborn babies. Although there is some controversy
here (some examples of various populations having relatively high
cholesterol levels but low CVD levels), this is a safe range to shoot for.
But as you will see, things are not as simple as one total number.

HDL Cholesterol
What Is That?

HDL is a form of lipoprotein that actually helps to move fats from the
peripheral body back to the liver. In digestive physiology, the liver is
literally the center of the universe. Food that is absorbed from the in-

testines is sent to the liver for processing, distributed throughout the body, and then brought back to the liver for reprocessing. This last part of the distribution process involves carrier molecules like HDL. HDLs are generally considered "good" cholesterol, as they appear to act as scrubbers in our arteries and veins, bringing fats back to the liver for processing. This notion is not entirely correct, but it's correct enough for our purposes.

How Much?

We are actually concerned with too little HDL cholesterol. Modern, sedentary populations show levels that are low due to consumption of trans fats and inadequate exercise. I'd like to see yours above 50 mg/dl.

LDL Cholesterol
What Is It?

LDL plays opposite HDL in the process of distributing lipid (fat) substances throughout the body. The energy we need to run our muscles, the raw material for our cell membranes, the omega-3 fats that make up our brain, are all shuttled around with the help of LDL (and chylomicrons for you geeks). LDL is generally considered the "bad" flavor of cholesterol, but as we will see, this is due to a myopic view of blood lipids in general and cholesterol in particular.

How Much?

Ancestral levels of LDL cholesterol appear to run in the range of 40–70mg/dl, but this is not the only consideration with LDL. We also have an issue of LDL particle size. Our LDL particles can come in a range of sizes from small and dense (called a "type B" profile) to large and puffy (called a "type A" profile)—and just so all the LDL particles feel good about themselves, the particles between small and large are considered "intermediate." Lipid scientists are nothing if they are not crafty with their names!

What does all this mean? It appears the type of LDL particle is of significantly greater importance than the amount. The type B profile, for example, appears to be particularly bad as the small, dense LDL particles get trapped in the nooks and crannies of the blood vessels. Our immune system is not used to seeing things get stuck in the gaps between cells in our blood vessels. Our immune system mistakes the small/dense LDL particles for a foreign invader and attacks them. This is the beginning of an atherosclerotic plaque, which can narrow key arteries such as the carotid artery. As you know, the carotid artery serves a fairly important organ—the brain. The coronary arteries that keep your ticker-ticking are also susceptible to blockage from atherosclerotic plaques. As the arteries narrow, your heart begins working less and less efficiently. This can progress until you have a really bad day: a small chunk of circulating schmootz plugs a narrowed artery in your heart or brain: heart attack or stroke.

Is this situation "luck-o-the-draw" with regard to what type of LDLs we have? Our medical establishment would have you believe it's only vaguely under dietary control. All the commercials about cholesterol-lowering drugs have an obligatory comment about "If diet and exercise does not change your condition, you might consider this drug." Cardiovascular disease can be easily controlled with diet and lifestyle changes—they just need to be the right changes!

Check This Out:

Type B LDLs are certainly atherogenic. Type A LDLs appear to be nonatherogenic. Type B (small, dense LDLs) are caused by *high insulin levels*. Our diet of choice (according to the American Heart Association) is a high-carb, low-fat diet. Hmmm. So, if you want to turn your LDL particles into nasty, highly reactive type Bs, you just need to eat a high-carb, grain-based diet! Now, what about the number of LDLs? How does diet affect that? Well, interestingly, high insulin levels increase total cholesterol production by up-regulating a key cholesterol synthesis enzyme called HMG-Co-a-Reductase. High insulin means not only small, dense cholesterol particles, but lots of them! Interestingly, glucagon reduces the activity of HMG-Co-A-Reductase. Do you see how all this stuff fits together?

So, when I put out that recommendation of 40–70 mg/dl of LDL cholesterol, we need to temper that with an awareness that LDL count is not nearly as compelling as the types of LDLs we have. Our medical establishment is still hyperfocused on the amount of cholesterol we have, yet people with low-medium cholesterol levels have heart attacks every day. If it was simply a numbers game, this should not happen.

The folks who have low numbers and CVD, tend to have dense, reactive particles and some other markers of systemic inflammation we will look at in a moment. When accurately assessing our cardiovascular risk factors, the bottom line with LDL cholesterol is we need to consider quality first (large or small particles) and quantity second.

Triglycerides
What Is It?

When we talk about dietary fats, we are actually talking about triglycerides. This is a molecule with three fatty acids (tri-) attached to a glycerol backbone. Triglycerides are a measure of circulating blood fats, so you would think a "high-fat diet" would mean high triglycerides, right? Interestingly, this is not the case. Triglycerides are in fact an indicator of dietary *carbohydrate* and insulin sensitivity. High carbs and poor insulin sensitivity = high triglycerides. Don't forget, excess dietary carbohydrate is converted to palmitic acid in the liver! Counterintuitively, excessive carbohydrate intake forms the backbone not only for most triglycerides but also small, dense, reactive LDL particles.

How Much?

Ancestral levels of triglycerides appear to be in the 50–80 mg/dl range. Triglycerides are, however, more the "canary in the coal-mine" than a direct cause of problems. If we have low triglycerides, we can be pretty sure we are not taking in too many dietary carbohydrates and our lifestyle issues are in order such that we are insulin sensitive. Conversely, if our triglycerides are above 100, we are likely to develop problems with inflammation and a shift toward the atherogenic blood profile predominated by small, dense LDL particles. Our clients routinely have triglycerides in the range of 30–40 mg with their other blood lipids following in lockstep. Oh, yeah—booze can create havoc with your triglycerides. If you are not particularly insulin sensitive, you need to go easy on the booze. Robb's Rule for Boozing: Drink enough to optimize your sex life, not so much that it impacts your blood lipids.

Hb1Ac (also goes by the alias "A1c")

The A1c has been one of my favorite lab values for years. It is a measure of how much sugar is sticking to your red blood cells. Since your red blood cells replace themselves every 120 days, this gives you a measure of your blood glucose levels over time. Folks with blood glucose management problems are encouraged to monitor blood glucose levels. This is helpful, but it provides a narrow slice of information. Blood glucose levels can be misleading in that they may be abnormally high or low at a given point due to stress, exercise, or other factors. The A1c is inexpensive, accurate, and tells us a ton of information. If your A1c level is above 5, you have big problems brewing. Your likelihood of CVD, cancer, and all the problems associated with elevated insulin levels is greatly elevated. I'd like to see your A1c level in the 4s. Keep in mind, if sugar is sticking to your red blood cells, it is also sticking to *all* the vital proteins in your body. This process, advanced glycation end products, appears to be the mechanism behind much of what we assume to be "normal" aging. Stiffness, loss of vision, and decreased kidney and brain function share AGEs as a causative mechanism. The A1c can tell us much about your nutrition, as well as your lifestyle. Inadequate sleep or other stressors that impair insulin sensitivity will manifest in elevated A1c, even if your nutrition is solid. I have recommended this biomarker in situations as different as cortisol management to gestational diabetes because of the amount of information obtained from this one measure.

C-Reactive Protein
What Is It?

C-reactive protein (CRP) is a *marker* of systemic inflammation. It is a by-product of immune cell activity and is not a problem itself, but rather an indicator of overall inflammation. If you have an infection, CRP will be elevated (hopefully), as you have immune cells battling the infection. This battle between your immune system and the infectious agent, be it viral, bacterial, fungal, or parasitic, causes an increase in CRP. What if you have elevated CRP but do not *appear* to have an infection? This may be an indicator of hidden inflammation in wacky places like the intestines or your gums. It is well understood that brushing and flossing is strongly correlated with decreased incidence of cardiovascular events. Why? Because dealing with gingivitis decreases systemic inflammation, which can increase one's likelihood of developing atherosclerotic lesions. Now consider that you have significantly more surface area in your intestines. What if they are inflamed from Neolithic foods, stress, and inadequate sleep? You can bet your CRP is elevated due to elevated immune activity and systemic inflammation.

How Much?
Healthy levels of CRP are below 1.0 mg/l. If you start with high numbers, altering your food and lifestyle should bring this number down.

Hypothetical Blood Work
Now that we have what to look for with regard to blood work, let's look at a hypothetical scenario so these numbers have some context. I will also look at the factors that are causing these numbers and how we might expect them to change with some smart nutrition and lifestyle changes.

Donny "DOA" Donnatelli

Donny is a forty-five-year-old business owner in Las Vegas. He travels frequently, as he must oversee the growth of his IT company. Donny rarely sleeps more than five hours per night, and he is driven and stressed. He is married, has three kids. He has not exercised in years, and his nutrition is rough by anyone's standards:

Breakfast:
Venti Caramel Macchiato with extra whip-cream, scone.

Snack:
Donny makes frequent rounds at the office, as there are numerous trays of cookies and pastries littered about.

Lunch:
Sandwich, soda, bag of chips, large cookie.

Dinner:
While his wife makes his favorite meal, spaghetti and meatballs, Donny "unwinds" with a martini or three. With his main course, he eats

toasted French bread with olive oil and consumes three glasses of wine. Tiramisu for dessert.

Donny has gained quite a bit of weight the past few years, but he is a big guy and has adjusted his wardrobe "up" when he needs new clothes. One day while trying to make a connection in the *worst* airport in the world, Phoenix Sky Harbor, Donny feels light headed and has some tightness in his chest. When he gets home, his wife guilts him into going to the doctor. His family doctor runs some standard blood work and refers him for a cardiac stress test. The cardiac stress test shows impaired heart function. Donny's blood work comes back the following:

Total cholesterol: 275
HDL 38
LDL 145
LDL particle size (predominantly type B, small, dense particles)
Triglycerides 300
A1c 5.8
Blood glucose 102
C-reactive protein 4.2 mg/l

Donny is lucky in that his doctor is a member of the Physician Network for Paleolithic Nutrition. His doc knows there is much more to the story than HDL/LDL. At Donny's follow-up, his doctor points out that in addition to Donny's poor performance on the cardiac stress test, he also has sleep apnea, serious acid reflux, and what might be gall-stones.

Donny's doctor lays it out: Donny will be lucky to see the age of fifty. He has a better chance to win the lottery than see age sixty. Without a serious overhaul, Donny's wife will be collecting his life insurance and retiring to Florida with Raul the pool boy. Donny likes the idea of that happening even less than dying, so he takes his doctors advice 100 percent—a grain-free, dairy-free, Paleo diet. He cuts back his travel schedule and starts delegating more tasks. He begins lifting weights a few days a week and walks on the other days. He guts the house and has nothing that is not fish, fowl, meat, fruit, veggies, or nuts in the pantry. The kids have a meltdown for a few days, then decide apples, oranges, almonds, and jerky are pretty damn tasty, especially when compared to starvation.

Six weeks later, Donny goes in for a checkup. He is down almost twenty-eight pounds and has removed four inches off his waist. His acid reflux and sleep apnea are "gone." His blood work has changed "a little":

Total cholesterol: 177
HDL 58
LDL 102
LDL particle size (mainly type A, large, nonreactive)
Triglycerides 84
A1c 5.1
Blood glucose 85
C-reactive protein 2.5 mg/l

This is very typical for a four- to eight-week change. Insulin levels plummeted due to a change in eating and lifestyle. Total cholesterol, triglycerides, and A1c dropped due to a decrease in dietary carbohydrates. HDL went up due to exercise and fish oil. Blood glucose is lower due to better overall diet, lower stress, and better insulin sensitivity. LDL particles have shifted to the large, puffy type A profile. With continued adherence to this program, these numbers would likely settle out in this neighborhood:

Total cholesterol: 153
HDL 58
LDL 78
LDL particle size (type A, large, nonreactive)
Triglycerides 45
A1c 4.6
Blood glucose 72
C-reactive protein 0.7 mg/dl

Is Donny's example extreme? Unfortunately, his previous lifestyle is all too common and is closer to the norm than not. Fortunately, however, his change is quite typical of someone who gives the program a legitimate shot. I have worked with dozens, if not hundreds, of "Donnys," and if they actually commit to the program, none find the sacrifice to be greater than the benefits: improved health and longer life.

How Often Should I Track Blood Work?

If you are sick and just beginning a program of nutrition and lifestyle changes, you should get a baseline before making any changes, run with things for a month, then retest. If you are sick or significantly overweight, I'd track blood work monthly for three to six months. This will give you a window into your change, and it offers nice support and motivation for your efforts. Once you reach a stable maintenance level, rechecking blood values once per year is fine, so long as your compliance is solid.

What If Things Are Not Working?

Are things going in the right direction? They should be, and if they are not, let's make the first point of evaluation one of honest self-reflection: Are you *really* doing the program 100 percent. Sleep, food, exercise? The folks we see who have "problems" in their blood work happen to be the same people who have "compliance issues." This stuff works, but only if you *do* it.

I've worked with enough people now to understand the trends clearly. Do some people tolerate more carbohydrate than others? Yes, so if we do not see triglycerides fall or LDL particle sizes change, and you are still eating a bunch of carbs, even if it's from "Paleo carbs" like fruit, we have an obvious place to look for a fix. Although we will look at different levels of compliance, if you have blood work that is in the danger zones, and you want that to change, do a grain-free, dairy-free Paleo diet, no exceptions. Sleep. Exercise. If you are not doing the program but hoping to garner the results, this is simply not realistic. Give the program a shot, get healthy, then decide if health and long life are actually worth the "sacrifices."

What about Statins?

Whenever blood work is discussed, statins are not far behind. The drugs were developed when we first thought cholesterol was the cause of CVD. They are designed to lower cholesterol with the idea being lower cholesterol = decreased CVD. Well, statins do lower cholesterol, and they also lower CVD risks for some people, but it has little to do with the cholesterol-lowering effects. When you dig a little deeper into the pharmacology of statins, you find they are anti-inflammatories. Unfortunately, however, statins also have some nasty side effects. If you have high cholesterol, your doctor will want to put you on statins. Your doctor is likely to think all this Paleo talk is unscientific prattle, so here is a deal you might try to broker with your doc:

Let you try this madness for thirty to sixty days. Track the above recommended blood work. Take some fish oil and a few other supplements we will look at later. If everything goes the direction it "should"—i.e., your systemic inflammation goes down, your LDL particles shift to the type A profile, your triglycerides plummet, your HDL goes up—maybe, just maybe, you do not need statins. That is ultimately up to you and your doctor to hash out, but if the main pharmacological action of statins is anti-inflammatory (it is), why is an anti-inflammatory lifestyle change not as good?

What If Things Are a Bit Different?

Occasionally, we have a client whose metabolism is just a bit different and the total cholesterol does not come down as much as they and their doctors might want. Is it time to panic or go wild with statins? I don't think so! Here's what I'd look at:

• CRP—If C-reactive protein is low, your systemic inflammation is likely low.
• LDL particle size should be large and puffy. If this is the case, things are looking good.
• A1c should be less than 5. If so, back away from the statins.
• Triglycerides are less than 50 mg. If your other biomarkers are in line, it's virtually a given this will be in line as well. If it's not, then it means we have some excess carbohydrate, stress, or a combination of the two.

What if all these biomarkers are just, well, close to being good? Well, how much do you enjoy living? If the biomarkers do not fall into place, you might have some genetic variability that makes your numbers a bit odd, and that may or may not mean a damn thing for your CVD risks. But this is rare. More often, these borderline numbers are proof you are a Cheater Mccheaterkins. Lack of compliance means lack of results, so be honest with yourself in this regard. It's just your life.

Here is all of the above information in one location. It includes the biomarker and recommended amounts or ranges, but remember, many of these items have a complex story associated with them.

Cholesterol total:	120–140 mg/dl
HDL cholesterol	>50 mg/dl
LDL cholesterol	40–70 mg/dl
Triglycerides	50–80 mg/dl
C-reactive protein	<1.0 mg/dl
Hb1Ac	<5

TWELVE

◇◇

Thirty-Day Meal Plan

◇◇

I'm pretty handy in the kitchen, but I wanted to bring in a different voice for the thirty-day meal plan. The first person I thought of was my good friend, strength coach and "underground" chef, Scott Hagnas. Scotty is not only one of the most knowledgeable coaches I know, he is also amazingly talented in the kitchen. Scotty has written a monthly Paleo Recipe column for the *Performance Menu* online journal for four years, and he has two amazing Paleo recipe books (*Cooking for Performance and Health* vols. 1 and 2, available at www.performancemenu. com).

The recipes in this thirty-day plan are for the most part simple. Every meal of every day cannot be a grand event. But the weekends get a little more involved, as these are the times you will hang out with friends and family and have a little more reason to "get fancy." You will notice that the breakfasts and lunches of many days are leftovers from the previous night's diner. That's called "planning ahead!"

Now that you have provisioned your home with the help of the shopping and food guide, you are ready to embark on your thirty-day Paleo challenge.

The following meal plans and recipes are merely suggestions. Feel free to modify them to suit your tastes and make use of what ingredients you have available. Having some go-to recipe basics will help you learn to create delicious meals on the fly using what ingredients you have on hand.

The snacks are optional. I have included them to help those who like to snack, but three good meals per day is fine. If you are serious about fat loss, you may wish to omit snacks or fruit.

Be sure to adjust the portion sizes as needed. Also, be sure to look ahead to see which recipes you'll want to prepare in large quantities for later use. Enjoy!

For menu items with an asterisk, refer to this week's cookbook for the recipe. The others require no other preparation.

Week 1

Monday
BREAKFAST: 2–4 poached eggs, almonds, small piece fruit or berries
LUNCH: Chicken Fajita Salad*
SNACK: 2 oz chicken, apple, few avocado slices
DINNER: Grilled Salmon*, Roasted Green Beans*, side salad

Tuesday
BREAKFAST: Leftover salmon, walnuts
LUNCH: Lettuce, tomato, onion, and condiments of your choice over 1–2 Burger Patties*, orange, almonds
SNACK: Jerky, macadamia nuts
DINNER: Rotisserie chicken, Steamed Broccoli*, side salad

Wednesday
BREAKFAST: Leftover chicken w/salsa, ½ avocado
LUNCH: Tuna and Cabbage Salad*
SNACK: Remainder of tuna and cabbage salad
DINNER: Crock-Pot Pork Loin, tomato sauce, zucchini, chopped cauliflower, basil. Make a large portion, leftovers will be used for several meals!

Thursday
BREAKFAST: Slice of ham, 2–3 scrambled eggs, fruit
LUNCH: Leftover pork loin
SNACK: 2 hard-boiled eggs, almonds
DINNER: Stir-Fry Beef Salad*. Serve over bed of greens with balsamic vinegar

Friday
BREAKFAST: Sausage Stir-Fry Breakfast*
LUNCH: Easy Ceviche*
SNACK: 2 oz chicken, apple
DINNER: Spaghetti Squash or Kelp Noodle Spaghetti*: cook either choice with marinara sauce, ground meat, olive oil

Saturday
BREAKFAST: Chicken Apple Hash*
LUNCH: 5–6 oz deli turkey, ½ lb steamed broccoli, drizzle with olive oil
SNACK: 2–3 oz turkey, carrot sticks, almonds
DINNER: Indian Style Slaw*, leftover pork loin, side salad with olive oil

Sunday
BREAKFAST: Western Omelet*, Sweet Potato Hash*
LUNCH: Lamb Patties*, tomato, lettuce, strawberries
SNACK: Turkey, avocado
DINNER: Halibut*, Roasted Asparagus*, berries with balsamic vinegar*

Week 1 Cookbook

Chicken Fajita Salad
- 1 tbsp olive oil
- ¾ cup sliced onions
- 1 lb skinless chicken breast
- ½ tsp cumin
- 2 tsp oregano
- 1 cup chopped bell peppers
- red leaf lettuce
- 1–2 tomatoes
- 1 avocado

Add olive oil to a skillet. Heat over medium. Add sliced onions, sauté until soft. Add the chicken, cut into strips. Add the cumin and oregano, sauté, tossing often. Add the bell peppers when the chicken has browned.

Wash and shred the lettuce. Add the tomatoes, toss. Serve the salad on two plates, top with the chicken fajita mix. Add the sliced avocado.

If you are taking this to work, assemble the salad into a container with a lid. Save some of the fajita mix for leftovers, use only ¼ to ⅓ of the chicken sauté for each of the salads you prepare.

Grilled Salmon

- coconut oil
- 1 lb salmon (wild-caught)
- 2 tbsp pecans
- 2 tsp rosemary
- sea salt

Preheat the oven to 350 degrees. Add a bit of coconut oil to a baking pan, coat well. Lay the salmon in the pan skin side down.

Chop the pecans. Sprinkle the pecans, rosemary, and sea salt over your fish, then bake for 12–15 minutes. Make sure it flakes easily with a fork; be sure to check the middle portion of the salmon.

Roasted Green Beans

- 1 lb green beans
- 1 tbsp olive oil
- 1 tbsp thyme

Chop the ends off of the beans. Place them into a roasting pan, add the olive oil and thyme. Toss until they are coated well, then roast in the oven at 350 degrees for 20 minutes. Check them occasionally, tossing several times.

Burger Patties

- 1 lb ground beef or turkey
- 1 tsp olive oil

Form the meat into 4 patties. We'll keep these simple, not adding eggs or spices, but you may do this if you like.

Add the oil to a skillet over medium heat, then cook the patties, turning often. Add the veggies and condiments of your choice.

Steamed Broccoli

- 1–2 lbs broccoli
- water

Cut the broccoli into individual florets. Add to your steamer basket, then add water to the bottom. Cover and cook over medium high until softened, around 8–10 minutes. Remove and serve.

Tuna and Cabbage Salad

- 3–4 cups shredded cabbage
- 1 can tuna (6.5 oz)
- 1 tbsp toasted sesame oil

Shred the cabbage into a bowl. Top with the tuna, drizzle with the oil.

Slow Cooker Pork Loin

- 3 lbs pork loin
- 1 can tomato sauce (12 oz)
- 2+ cups sliced zucchini
- 4 cups chopped cauliflower florets
- 1–2 tbsp basil

Add all of the ingredients to a large Crock-Pot. Cook on low for 6–7 hours, then enjoy.

Stir-Fry Beef Salad

- 2 tsp olive oil
- ¾ cup sliced onion
- 1 lb beef tip steak, sliced into thin strips
- 1 tbsp wheat-free tamari soy sauce
- 1–2 cups sliced bell peppers
- 1 bag of mixed greens
- balsamic vinegar

Add olive oil to a skillet. Heat over medium. Add sliced onions, sauté until soft. Add the beef and the tamari, tossing often. Add the bell peppers when the beef has browned.

To save time, use a bag of mixed greens. Add to your plates, then top with the stir fry meat. Add balsamic vinegar and more olive oil to taste.

Sausage Stir-Fry Breakfast

- 1–2 tsp olive oil
- ½ cup diced onions
- ½ lb sausages, sliced (no nitrates)
- 4 cups of spinach or other greens

Add olive oil to a skillet. Heat over medium. Add diced onions, sauté until soft. Add the sausage, cook until browned, tossing occasionally. Add the greens, reduce the heat to medium-low and cover. Serve when the greens are wilted and soft.

Other options: top with 1–2 eggs over easy, or serve with salsa.

Easy Ceviche

- 10 oz tail-off, precooked shrimp
- 2 cups low-sugar marinara sauce
- 2 tbsp olive oil
- 2 tbsp lemon juice
- 1 tsp basil

Rinse the shrimp, divide between two bowls. Pour half of the marinara sauce over each bowl of shrimp, then drizzle each with 1 tbsp of both olive oil and lemon juice. Sprinkle with the basil. Enjoy!

Spaghetti

- 1 lb ground beef or turkey
- 1 tbsp olive oil
- 1 (12 oz) package of kelp noodles, or one spaghetti squash
- 1–2 cups marinara sauce
- 1–2 cloves crushed garlic

Brown the meat in the olive oil using a large skillet. Once the meat is browned, add the noodles (or cooked spaghetti squash, see below) and the marinara sauce. Stir and bring to a simmer. Add the crushed garlic just before serving to maximize the health benefits.

If using spaghetti squash: Preheat the oven to 375 degrees. Carefully split the squash lengthwise, then dig out the seeds. Place both halves face down on a baking pan, add ¼ cup of water. Bake for 30 minutes. Dig out the squash with a fork and add to your skillet with the meat.

Chicken Apple Hash

- 2 tsp olive oil
- 6 oz leftover chicken
- 1 apple
- 2 tsp either cinnamon or allspice (choose your favorite)

Heat the olive oil in a saucepan over medium heat. Shred and add the chicken. Grate the apple, then add to the pot with your spice of choice. Cover and cook on medium-low, stirring frequently. Once the apple has cooked down and become soft, it is ready to serve.

Indian-Style Slaw

Here is an easy, cheap veggie idea. If you use a bag of ready-made broccoli slaw, you can really save time. Tomatoes are optional. Though this is a stand-alone veggie dish, you could add some leftover meat to this for a complete meal.

- 1 tbsp olive oil
- 1 tsp mustard seeds
- 1 bag broccoli slaw
- 1 cup fresh diced tomatoes (optional)
- 1 tsp cumin
- ¼ tsp turmeric
- 2 tbsp lemon juice

Heat 1 tbsp of olive oil over medium heat in a skillet, add 1 tsp of mustard seeds. Cover and cook until the seeds stop popping. Next, add the whole bag of slaw, the tomatoes (if using), plus 1 tsp cumin and ¼ tsp of turmeric. Sauté for 3–5 minutes, tossing occasionally, until the slaw is soft. Add 2 tbsp of lemon juice. Stir and serve.

Western Omelet
- 6 eggs
- olive oil
- ⅓ cup chopped onion
- ⅓ cup chopped bell peppers
- ½ cup chopped tomato
- 1 cup spinach
- 4 oz diced ham
- sea salt and black pepper to taste

Crack all of the eggs into a bowl, beat well. Pour half of the eggs into a nonstick skillet coated with a dash of olive oil. Cook over medium. When the eggs have begun to set, add half the chopped veggies and ham to one side of the eggs. Using a spatula, fold the empty half over the ham and veggies. Cook for 1–2 minutes longer, season with salt and pepper, then serve. Repeat the process with the remaining ingredients.

Sweet Potato Hash
- 2 tsp olive oil
- ½ cup chopped onions
- 1 medium sweet potato or yam, diced into small cubes
- ½ cup chopped bell peppers (optional)
- 1 tbsp water
- fresh ground pepper

Heat the oil in a skillet over medium heat. Add the onions, sauté for 2–3 minutes. Add the sweet potatoes and bell peppers and 1 tbsp of water. Cover and cook for 15 minutes or until the potatoes are soft. Toss often to prevent burning. Serve, sprinkling with fresh ground pepper.

Lamb Patties
Simply prepare these the same as Beef Patties above, using ground lamb instead.

Halibut
- 1 lb halibut or other white fish
- 2 tbsp chopped almonds

• 2 tbsp Dijon mustard

Prepare in the same fashion as the baked salmon above, except season by spreading Dijon mustard and chopped almonds over your fish.

Roasted Asparagus
• 1 bunch asparagus
• 1 tbsp olive oil
• 2 tsp thyme

Break the tough ends off of the asparagus. Place in a roasting pan, pour the oil and thyme over the asparagus, then toss until well coated.

Bake at 400 degrees for 10 minutes, then reduce the heat to 250 for 15 more minutes.

Berries with Balsamic Vinegar
• 2 cups frozen berry mix, thawed
• 4 tsp balsamic vinegar

Divide the berries between two bowls. Pour two teaspoons of balsamic vinegar over each. A simple, nutritious dessert! Fresh berries will be even better if you have the time to prepare them.

Week 2

Monday
BREAKFAST: Slice of ham, 1 cup unsweetened applesauce w/cinnamon, 1 oz walnuts
LUNCH: Make a big salad: toss chicken strips, lettuce, olives, tomato, chopped almonds, and carrot strips. Add olive oil and vinegar of your choice.
SNACK: Pack extra salad; save ⅓ of the lunch salad for your snack if you want one
DINNER: Tip Steak* and Steamed Vegetables*

Tuesday

BREAKFAST: Leftover steak, 1–2 oz macadamia nuts
LUNCH: Chicken Breast*, Indian-Style Slaw*
SNACK: Leftovers from lunch, plums
DINNER: Pork Curry*

Wednesday

BREAKFAST: Slice of ham, unsweetened applesauce, spoon of almond butter
LUNCH: Leftover tip steak, sliced into strips. Serve on salad of mixed greens, tomato, bell pepper, balsamic vinegar, and olive oil.
SNACK: Jerky, ½ avocado
DINNER: Leftover pork curry, Chilled Cucumber Soup*

Thursday

BREAKFAST: Ginger Eggs*
LUNCH: Beet Apple Salad*, Tilapia*
SNACK: Jerky, ½ avocado
DINNER: Chicken and Cauliflower*

Friday

BREAKFAST: 2–3 eggs over easy, served over Sautéed Zucchini*
LUNCH: Smoked Turkey Salad*
SNACK: Jerky and macadamia nuts
DINNER: Quick Chicken Curry*

Saturday

BREAKFAST: Slice of ham, Quick Paleo Pancakes*
LUNCH: Rotisserie chicken, steamed veggies of your choice (such as broccoli, cauliflower, carrots)
SNACK: Leftover chicken curry
DINNER: Lamb Sausage with Artichokes*

Sunday

BREAKFAST: Peach 'n' Pecan Scramble*, leftover chicken
LUNCH: Burger, no bun, over greens, side salad
SNACK: Orange, leftover meat or tuna, celery or carrot sticks
DINNER: Paleo Chicken Alfredo*

Week 2 Cookbook

Tip Steak
• 4 lb tip steak
• seasonings of your choice

Bring a skillet to medium heat, add a dash of olive oil. Season the steak, then cook it to your desired doneness. I like to cook the meat just a couple of minutes per side, then plate and cover for 10 minutes. Remember that cooking too long with excessive browning or burning creates carcinogens!

Steamed Vegetables
• 4 cups chopped cauliflower florets
• 2 cups sliced yellow squash
• 1 cup sliced carrots
• olive oil
• sea salt and pepper
• 1 tsp thyme

Chop the vegetables. Add to your steamer basket, then add water to the bottom. Cover and cook over medium high until softened, around 8–10 minutes. Remove and serve. Drizzle with olive oil, and add salt, pepper, and thyme to taste

Chicken Breast
• 2 lbs chicken breasts, thawed

Place the chicken in a baking dish, bake at 350 degrees until done—around 25 minutes. Check to ensure your meat has been cooked all the way through, but be careful not to overcook as well. Have some for lunch, save the leftovers for use later.

Indian-Style Slaw
Refer to Week 1 Cookbook

Pork Curry

- 1 lb ground pork
- 1 tbsp olive oil
- 1–2 tbsp curry powder
- 1 bag baby spinach (~14 oz)
- ½ can coconut milk (7 oz)
- 2–3 cloves garlic

In a pot large enough to hold the spinach, brown the pork in the olive oil. Add the curry powder as the pork browns, mix well. Break up any large lumps of pork. Once the pork has browned, add all of the spinach and the coconut milk. Heat until the spinach has cooked down and wilted. Add the garlic at the end, either mincing it or using a garlic press to crush it. Mix well, remove from heat, and serve.

This recipe works well with stew beef, chicken, or lamb as well.

Beet Apple Salad

- 1 lb beets
- 2 tbsp olive oil
- 2 tbsp lemon juice
- 1 apple
- ½ cup finely chopped red onion
- ½ to 1 tsp tarragon

Cut the tops off of the beets, then place them in a pot and cover with water. Cover and simmer over medium-low heat for 1¼ hours. Allow the beets to cool.

Drain the beets, cut off the root, and peel the skin. Slice the beets crosswise into thin slices, then place them in a bowl. Pour the oil and lemon juice over the beets, then chill in the refrigerator.

Core and chop the apple. Chop the onion. Mix into the beets, sprinkle some tarragon on top, and serve.

Tilapia

- 2 tsp olive oil
- ½ tsp lemon peel
- garlic powder to taste

- onion powder to taste
- 1½ lbs tilapia fillets

Heat the oil in a skillet over medium heat. Add the lemon peel and spices to the tilapia fillets. Cook the fish, turning once, until it flakes easily with a fork. Remove some to a container, preferably ceramic, to bring with you for lunch. Save the rest for an easy dinner.

Chilled Cucumber Soup

- 2 medium cucumbers
- ½ cup chopped onion
- ¼ cup fresh cilantro leaves
- ½ cup coconut milk
- ¼ cup chicken broth

Peel the cucumber, then chop it into small chunks. Load the onion, cucumber, and cilantro into your blender. Add the coconut milk and chicken broth. Blend until smooth, but not too fine. Refrigerate, then serve cold. Garnish with some more cilantro.

Makes 4 servings

Ginger Eggs

- 1 tsp chili oil
- ½ cup green beans
- 1 tbsp minced ginger
- 1 small clove garlic, minced
- 3 eggs
- 1 tbsp chopped chives or green onions
- ¼ tsp coriander
- pepper to taste

Heat the oil in a small skillet. Add the green beans, sauté for 2 minutes. Add the ginger and garlic, cook 3 minutes more. Meanwhile, crack the eggs into a bowl, whip well. Add the beans, ginger, and garlic, plus the chives or onions and coriander. Mix well, then return to the skillet. Cook until the eggs set. Serve topped with fresh ground pepper.

Smoked Turkey Salad

- 10 oz smoked turkey (from the deli section)
- 1 bag mixed greens
- ¼ cup pine nuts

You can mix this dish and then store it in the refrigerator. Make sure to thoroughly rinse the greens.

Chicken and Cauliflower

Here is a quick one-pot meal. You can also prepare this one in a slow cooker, simply add the same ingredients and set to low. If you choose this route, the cooking time will be around 5 hours.

We have frequently sung the praises of El Pato tomato sauce. For this recipe, I use the milder version that comes in the red can. Check the Hispanic foods section of your grocery store for El Pato. If you can't find it, any good tomato sauce will work.

- 1 tbsp olive oil
- 1½ lbs chicken thighs or breast
- 1 head of cauliflower
- 8 oz tomato sauce (El Pato with jalapeño)
- 1 red bell pepper
- 1 tsp cumin
- 1 tsp thyme
- ½ tsp garlic powder

Heat the olive oil over medium heat in either a large skillet or soup pot. Brown the chicken on all sides. Meanwhile, chop the cauliflower into small pieces and add to the pot. Add all of the remaining ingredients to the pot, then reduce to medium-low. Cover and cook for 45 minutes, stirring occasionally.

Makes 5 servings

Sautéed Zucchini

- 2 small zucchini
- ¼ cup either sliced shallots or red onion
- 2 cloves garlic, sliced

- 2 tbsp olive oil
- dill
- pepper

Slice the zucchini crosswise into small discs about ¼ inch thick. Slice the shallots or onion and garlic.

Sauté all of the ingredients together in a medium pan with the olive oil. Add dill and pepper to taste. Stir and turn often, cooking for 5 to 7 minutes. Try not to allow too much browning. Enjoy warm, or these can be used cold in salads.

Quick Chicken Curry

Pressed for time, you can make use of curry sauce. Look in better markets for curry sauces that are made from quality ingredients and do not contain added sugars. An alternative is to use coconut milk and a teaspoon of yellow curry paste.

You can either use fresh or leftover chicken with this recipe.

- ½ cup chopped onion
- 1 tbsp olive oil
- 1 diced chicken breast or thigh
- ¼ cup curry sauce
- ¼ cup cashews
- 2 cups chopped spinach

Sauté the onion in the olive oil until translucent. Add chicken, heat until cooked through. Add the curry sauce and cashews, continue heating for 3–4 minutes. Remove from heat, stir in the spinach.

Quick Paleo Pancakes

Here is a way to enjoy pancakes while avoiding using grains.

- 2 eggs
- ½ cup unsweetened applesauce
- ½ cup nut butter (not peanut butter! - cashew/macadamia nut butter works well)
- ¼ tsp cinnamon

- ¼ tsp vanilla extract
- coconut oil

Mix all of the ingredients except the coconut oil in a bowl. Stir well, until you have a uniform batter. Next, use a bit of coconut oil to grease a non-stick skillet. Spread some of the batter into the skillet to form a pancake, then cook over low/medium heat. Flip after 1 to 2 minutes, being careful not to burn them!

Once you've cooked all of your pancakes, you can serve them with a variety of toppings. A few that I like: chopped apples and cinnamon; heated blueberries; real maple syrup; and unsweetened applesauce.

Lamb Sausage with Artichokes

This is a simple, delicious breakfast. Don't worry if you can't find Moroccan lamb sausages anywhere. Simply use some sausages of your choice, then add some Moroccan spices. Moroccan seasonings include cinnamon, coriander, allspice, ginger, and cloves. Try adding any combination of these spices—about ⅛ tsp of each.

- 1 oz bacon, chopped
- 2 Moroccan lamb sausages, sliced
- 1 (14 oz) can artichoke hearts (Trader Joe's)
- 1–2 omega-3 eggs
- sea salt to taste
- fresh ground pepper to taste

Chop the bacon, place in a skillet over medium heat. Meanwhile, slice the sausage and chop the artichoke hearts. Once the bacon has softened, add the sausage and artichokes. If using the spices, add them at this point. Stir well, cooking until soft.

Poach your eggs in the meantime. Cover the bottom of a skillet with about 1 inch of water, then place over medium heat. Once the water is warm, crack your eggs carefully into the skillet, cook until set.

Serve the artichoke hash topped with either 1 or 2 eggs. Add sea salt and fresh ground pepper to taste.

Peach and Pecan Scramble

This is a very unusual combination, but it is surprisingly delicious. It's almost like dessert at breakfast, and way better for you than stopping by the donut shop!

I've written this recipe as a one-person snack or light breakfast; increase the quantities if you like.

- 1 tsp olive oil
- ½ peach, diced
- 2 tbsp chopped pecans
- 2 eggs
- 1 tbsp unsweetened applesauce
- ⅛ tsp cinnamon

Heat the olive oil in a small skillet over medium heat. Dice half of a ripe peach, and chop the pecans. Add the peaches and pecans to the skillet, stir-fry for 2–3 minutes, or until the peaches soften a bit.

Meanwhile, crack the eggs into a bowl, add the applesauce and cinnamon, and beat well. Add to the skillet, mixing often. When the eggs have set, serve and enjoy.

Paleo Chicken Alfredo

Alfredo sauce and pasta is about as far from Paleo nutrition as you can get. However, here is a simple way to create a Paleo version. I am using kelp noodles here, but if you cannot find them where you live, spaghetti squash is a nice seasonal alternative. See the Week 1 Spaghetti recipe above for basic spaghetti squash preparation.

- 2 tsp olive oil
- 4 cloves of garlic, chopped
- 1 lb chicken breast
- 1 (12 oz) package of kelp noodles
- 2 tsp tarragon
- 1 cup cashews
- ½ tsp onion powder
- ¼ tsp garlic powder
- ¼ tsp mustard powder

- ¼ tsp sea salt
- ¼ tsp pepper
- ⅛ tsp paprika

Add the olive oil to a large skillet. Sauté the garlic over medium heat for 3–4 minutes. Chop the chicken into 1 inch cubes, then add to the skillet and cook until browned on all sides.

Rinse and chop the kelp noodles. Add them to the skillet along with the tarragon, cover and cook on low for 30 minutes. Then, pour the liquid from the skillet carefully into a small container for use in the sauce.

Add the cashews, onion powder, garlic powder, mustard powder, salt, pepper, and paprika to a blender. Cover and blend into a powder. Add the reserved pan juices slowly, blending into a thick sauce. You'll have to use a spatula to scrape down the sides of the blender periodically. Add the juices until the mixture reaches the desired consistency.

Add the sauce to the skillet, then mix well. Cover and continue to cook for 10 minutes longer, until the kelp noodles have become tender.

Week 3

Monday
BREAKFAST: Boiled lamb sausage, apple
LUNCH: Leftover Paleo Chicken Alfredo
SNACK: Lamb sausage, pecans
DINNER: Spaghetti-Sauced Meat over Green Beans*

Tuesday
BREAKFAST: Boiled lamb sausage, apple (reheat on the stove, not microwave)
LUNCH: Chicken Apple Salad*
SNACK: Leftover spaghetti
DINNER: Slow-Cooked Rosemary Veggies and Meat*

Wednesday
BREAKFAST: Bacon, 2–3 eggs over easy or poached
LUNCH: Leftover Chicken Apple Salad

SNACK: Leftover Slow-Cooked Rosemary Veggies and Meat
DINNER: Flank steak, Bacon and Greens*

Thursday
BREAKFAST: Leftover steak, walnuts crumbled over ½ cup berries
LUNCH: Leftover Slow-Cooked Rosemary Veggies and Meat
SNACK: Can of sardines, celery
DINNER: Salmon Scramble*

Friday
BREAKFAST: Boiled quality sausages (chicken-apple sausages are delicious), Fruit Salad with Cinnamon*
LUNCH: Salad: mixed greens, bell peppers, tomato, avocado, etc. Top with precooked shrimp, apple cider vinegar, and olive oil
SNACK: Remainder of the lunch salad (make enough!)
DINNER: Sloppy Joes*, side salad or steamed veggies

Saturday
BREAKFAST: Poached eggs with bacon, onion, and spinach
LUNCH: Leftover Sloppy Joes
SNACK: Almonds
DINNER: Baked 1 turkey breasts, Nutty Cabbage*, Tangy Strawberry Soup*

Sunday
BREAKFAST: Turkey/Carrot Quiche*
LUNCH: Leftover turkey, Chard and Cashew Sauté*
SNACK: Lunch leftovers
DINNER: Jambalaya*

Week 3 Cookbook

Spaghetti-Sauced Meat
over Roasted Green Beans

- 3 lbs ground beef (grass-fed if possible), turkey, or chicken
- ½ cup chopped onions
- 2–3 cloves minced garlic
- 1 6 oz can tomato paste
- 1 20 oz can tomato sauce
- 2 tsp oregano
- 2 tsp basil
- 1 tsp tarragon
- 2+ lbs frozen green beans (or fresh)
- olive oil

Start cooking the ground meat in a large skillet over medium heat. If the meat is frozen, browning will take 8–10 minutes. Once the meat has been browned, add onions and fresh garlic. Then add 1 can of tomato paste, 1 can tomato sauce, oregano, basil, and tarragon, then cover with a lid for 20 minutes.

While the spaghetti meat is cooking, throw some frozen green beans onto a broiler pan, toss with olive oil and broil (making sure to stir green beans frequently). After about 5–8 minutes, the green beans should be slightly crispy.

Plate the green beans; top with the meat sauce. Add salt and pepper to taste.

Chicken Apple Salad

- 6 oz chicken
- 1 tsp olive oil
- ½ tsp allspice
- ⅛ tsp cloves
- 6 cups shredded cabbage
- ½ Granny Smith apple
- sea salt and pepper to taste

Dice the chicken. Heat 1 tsp of olive oil in a skillet over medium heat. Add the chicken, allspice, and cloves. Sauté, tossing often, until the chicken is cooked through.

Shred the cabbage into a large salad bowl. Slice half of an apple into very thin slices and set them aside.

Once the chicken is done, add it to the cabbage, then top with the apple. Add salt and pepper to taste, then drizzle with olive oil. Use an appropriate quantity of olive oil to meet your individual needs.

Slow-Cooked Rosemary Veggies and Meat

- 3–5 lbs any meat, frozen or thawed, ground or whole (fish is not usually ideal here).
- 1 bag frozen veggies or chopped-up fresh veggies.
- 1 tbsp rosemary
- 1 cup broth (chicken, beef, or vegetable)
- salt and pepper to taste

Add all of the ingredients to a slow cooker, turn to low and leave for 6–8 hours or until ready to eat.

Bacon and Greens

You can use fresh veggies, or if you want to save time, a bag of Trader Joe's Southern Greens works great here.

- 4–6 oz chopped bacon
- 1 12-16 oz bag Southern Greens, or 1 bunch each of collard greens, turnip greens, and/or kale
- ½ cup water
- sea salt and pepper to taste.

Chop the bacon and add to a large stockpot. Heat over medium, stirring the bacon until it has browned some. Add the greens and water, cover and reduce to medium-low. Cook for 30 minutes, tossing occasionally.

Some options to spice it up: add garlic, red pepper flakes, even minced jalapeños while browning the bacon. Another cooking option is to prepare this in a slow cooker.

Salmon Scramble

- 1 lb package frozen veggies
- 1 can salmon (6oz)
- 1 tbsp rosemary
- 1 tsp cumin
- 1 tsp sea salt
- pepper to taste
- eggs (optional)

Place frozen veggies in a saucepan with a lid, cook until just tender. Add salmon and seasonings cook another 3–5 minutes, mixing, until salmon is heated thoroughly. You can cook eggs sunny side up to top this scramble. If you don't have eggs, this is still great to eat plain. (This recipe also works with nearly all types of meat)

Fruit Salad with Cinnamon

- 1 orange, peeled and chopped
- 1 apple, chopped
- ½ tsp cinnamon

Place the fruit into bowls, then sprinkle with the cinnamon if you wish.

Sloppy Joes

Here is a spicy cocoa version of an old favorite. Since we will not be serving this on the traditional hamburger bun, you have several options. I like to make a bed of romaine lettuce and tomato slices, but there are many possibilities: eggplant, squash, nut patties, you name it.

- 1½ lbs ground turkey or beef (preferably grass-fed)
- 1 cup chopped onion
- 1 cup tomato puree
- 2 tbsp cocoa powder
- 1 tbsp chili powder
- ½ tsp yellow mustard powder
- 1½ tsp ground black pepper

Cook meat and onion in a large skillet on medium heat for 10–15 minutes, until the meat is browned. Stir in the remaining ingredients and heat for another 10–15 minutes. Serve over vegetables of your choice. Makes 4 servings.

Nutty Cabbage

- ½ cup chopped onions
- 1 tbsp roasted hazelnut oil
- ½ large head of cabbage, shredded (about 10 cups)
- ¼ cup apple cider vinegar
- ¼ cup blanched almonds
- 1 tbsp unsweetened applesauce
- 1 tbsp sesame seeds
- sea salt and fresh ground pepper to taste

Heat a burner to medium, then use a large skillet to sauté the onions in the oil. Meanwhile, shred the cabbage by slicing it thinly. After the onions begin to soften, add all of the cabbage to the skillet, along with the vinegar. Cover and reduce the heat to medium-low. Cook for 20 minutes, mixing occasionally. Add the remaining ingredients and cook 5 minutes longer. Serve warm or chilled.

Tangy Strawberry Soup

- 1 quart strawberries
- 4 tbsp balsamic vinegar, divided
- ½ tsp cinnamon
- ½ tsp orange zest
- ½ tsp lemon zest
- 1 tbsp orange juice
- ½ cup coconut milk

Remove the stems from all of the strawberries. Reserve 10–20 strawberries; cut these berries into thin slices. Place in a bowl, then drizzle with 2 tbsp of balsamic vinegar. Cover and chill in the refrigerator for two hours.

Puree the rest of the strawberries in a blender with the remaining ingredients except the coconut milk (adding only the remaining 2 tbsp of balsamic vinegar). Once the berry mix is pureed, add the coconut milk slowly. Puree until smooth. Pour the soup into a bowl, cover and chill in the fridge for 2 hours.

Serve in small bowls with the sliced strawberries on top. You can add a dollop of coconut milk for added garnish, if you like!

Turkey Carrot Quiche

- ½ lb ground turkey
- 1 tbsp olive oil
- 1 cup shredded carrots
- 6 omega-3 eggs
- 5 tbsp coconut milk
- ½ cup beef broth
- 4 tbsp fresh parsley
- ½ tsp coriander
- coconut oil

Brown the turkey in a bit of olive oil in a skillet over medium heat. Meanwhile, shred the carrots.

Crack the eggs into a bowl; beat well with a wire whip. Add the meat when done, carrots, and all of the remaining ingredients except the coconut oil. Stir.

Grease a baking dish or pie pan with some coconut oil. Pour in the mixture, then bake at 250 degrees for 20–30 minutes. You will need to check on it periodically; it is done when the center is firm and a knife pushed into it comes out clean.

Chard and Cashew Sauté

- 1 bunch Swiss chard
- 1 tbsp olive oil
- ½ cup cashews

Remove the stems from the chard, then chop the stems crosswise. Add to a large skillet with the olive oil. Sauté over medium heat until they have softened.

Meanwhile, chop the chard leaves into thin strips. Add to the skillet along with the cashews. Sauté, tossing occasionally, until the leaves just begin to wilt. Serve warm.

Jambalaya

This one is a spicy Southern dish. I use El Pato sauce, but if you are not a fan of spicy foods, you might consider regular tomato sauce instead. Look for sausages that don't contain nitrates.

- 1 tbsp olive oil + 1 tsp, divided
- ½ lb spicy sausage, sliced (look for andouille sausage)
- 1 cup chopped onion
- ¾ cup chopped green pepper
- ½ cup chopped celery
- 1 tsp Cajun seasoning + ⅛ tsp, divided
- 1 bay leaf
- 2 small cans El Pato tomato sauce
- 2 cups chicken broth
- 1½ cups water
- 1½ cups finely chopped cauliflower
- dash of cayenne pepper
- ½ lb shrimp

In a large skillet, heat the olive oil, sausage, onion, peppers, and celery. Sauté for around 5 minutes, then add the seasoning and bay leaf. Cook for 1 minute more. Add the tomato sauce, chicken broth, water, and cauliflower. Bring to a boil, then cover, reduce heat to medium-low, and simmer for 20 minutes. Remove the bay leaf.

In another skillet, sauté ½ lb of shrimp, ⅛ tsp Cajun seasoning, and a dash of cayenne pepper in 1 tsp olive oil. Sauté for 2 minutes, then stir into the jambalaya.

Week 4

Monday
BREAKFAST: Hard-boiled eggs, almonds, ½ cup berries
LUNCH: Tuna and cabbage salad
SNACK: Easy Ceviche
DINNER: Portobello Burgers*, steamed broccoli

Tuesday
BREAKFAST: Hard-boiled eggs, crushed walnuts over ½ cup berries
LUNCH: Leftover Portobello Burgers
SNACK: Deli turkey, ½ avocado
DINNER: Baked pork loin, Steamed Seasonal Veggies*

Wednesday
BREAKFAST: Leftover pork loin, egg, applesauce
LUNCH: Salad: turkey over spinach, walnuts, few dried cranberries, balsamic vinegar, olive oil
SNACK: Turkey, ½ avocado
DINNER: Pork and Roasted Veggie Salad*

Thursday
BREAKFAST: Sausage Stir Fry Breakfast
LUNCH: Leftover Pork and Roasted Veggie Salad
SNACK: Almond butter on celery sticks
DINNER: Curried Veggies with Salmon

Friday
BREAKFAST: Chicken Apple Hash, or leftover chicken + apple
LUNCH: Delicata Squash Salad*, steak
SNACK: 2 hard-boiled eggs, carrots
DINNER: Almond Chicken*

Saturday
BREAKFAST: Squash and Pepper Hash*, large slice of ham
LUNCH: Tuna and Cabbage Salad
SNACK: Jicama slices, salsa, guacamole
DINNER: Paleo Pizza*

Sunday
BREAKFAST: Egg Torte, ham
LUNCH: Tip Steak, Chilled Cucumber Soup*
DINNER: Greek Scallops*, side salad

Week 4 Cookbook

Portobello Burgers

Portobello mushrooms can make good substitutes for hamburger buns.
I just use one mushroom for the bottom "bun," but you could use two if
you'd like it to look a bit more traditional.

Time: 20–25 minutes

- 1 lb ground buffalo (or beef, turkey, etc.)
- ¼ cup chopped onion
- 2–3 cloves chopped garlic
- dash of pepper
- 1 tbsp olive oil
- 6 slices tomato
- lettuce
- 3 portobello mushrooms

Put the ground meat into a bowl, add the onion, garlic, pepper, and any
other spices that you wish. Mix well, then form into three patties. Place
the olive oil in a skillet, cook the patties, flipping often, until done to your
liking. I like to flip the meat often to prevent any excessive browning, and
serve it done rare. Set the burgers aside when done, covering with a plate
so that they stay warm.

While the burgers are cooking, prepare the "buns" and any vegetables
that you wish to top the burgers with. You'll want to cut the stems out of
the mushrooms first, but you can save them to use in a different meal if
you wish. Garnish your burgers any way you like.

Place the mushrooms into the skillet that you used to cook the burgers and cook for around 2–3 minutes per side in the juices from the meat.
Plate the mushrooms, then add the meat and condiments of your choos-
ing. A bit of steamed broccoli can round out this particular meal.

Seasonal Steamed Vegetables

- 1 medium zucchini, diced
- 1 medium yellow summer squash, diced
- 1 stalk broccoli florets, chopped into bite-sized pieces

- 2 cups spinach
- 2 slices of red onion
- 2 tbsp olive oil or coconut oil
- ½ tsp thyme
- sea salt to taste

Chop the vegetables. To save time, add water to your steamer and bring it to a boil while you are chopping the veggies. Add the vegetables to the basket, then reduce the heat and steam for around 10 minutes, or until the vegetables have reached the desired softness.

Serve the vegetables drizzled with either olive oil or coconut oil. I use 2 tbsp in this recipe, but be sure to adjust the amount to suit your own needs. Sprinkle with thyme and sea salt.

You can use many other vegetables in this recipe. Just be aware that some vegetables, such as cabbage, will take longer to steam. Add them to the steamer first, then add the other vegetables later for best results.

Pork and Roasted Veggie Salad

- 1 cup roasted yam and sweet potato mix
- ¾ cup roasted zucchini
- ¾ cup roasted asparagus
- olive oil
- seasonings of your choice (see below)
- 6 cups of herb salad mix
- 10 oz leftover pork loin
- sea salt to taste
- pepper to taste

First, roast your veggies.* Chop the yam and sweet potatoes into small cubes. Slice the zuchs into ¼-inch-thick discs, and break off the woody ends of the asparagus. Toss all of the veggies onto a roasting pan, drizzle with olive oil. Add any seasonings that you like here. I use red pepper flakes, but smoked paprika would be a good choice as well. If you avoid nightshades, basil is tasty. Toss until they are coated in the oil, then roast in the oven for 20 minutes at 350 degrees. Toss occasionally; when all of the veggies have become soft and slightly browned, they are done.

Make a bed of greens on two plates. To save time, you can use a pre-made herb greens mix. Top with the meat and roasted veggies. You can first warm the leftover meat in the oven if you like, or just add it cold. Top with sea salt and fresh ground pepper to taste.

* I suggest roasting a big batch, so that you have some left for later uses.

Curry Veggies

- 1 bag frozen veggies (or better yet, fresh)
- ½ 12-16 oz can coconut milk
- 1 cup chicken or beef broth
- 1 6-12 oz can of salmon or 1 lb of meat of your choice
- 1 tsp curry
- 1 tsp cumin
- 1 tsp garlic powder

Lightly steam frozen veggies until crisp-tender. Pour ½ can of coconut milk into a saucepan. Add the veggies, protein, and remaining spices. Mix all ingredients together and cook about 10 minutes to allow flavors to infuse. (This also can be a great slow cooker recipe and easily be doubled or tripled for planning ahead)

You may also substitute any variety of meats you prefer.

Delicata Squash Salad

- 1 Delicata squash
- 3½ tbsp olive oil (divided)
- sea salt (optional)
- 8 cups veggies: mix of Lacinato kale, curly kale, chard, radicchio, frisée.
- 2 tsp lemon juice
- 1 tsp Dijon mustard
- 2 tsp balsamic vinegar
- 1 tsp lemon peel
- 2 tbsp pine nuts

Preheat your oven to 350 degrees. Cut the squash in half lengthwise, then scoop out the seeds. Chop the squash into cubes, then toss with 2 tbsp of olive oil in a roasting pan. Sprinkle with sea salt if you like. Roast for 30 minutes, tossing every 10 minutes or so.

Meanwhile, chop your veggies, then toss them in a large salad bowl. I use a wide variety of seasonal greens, but your salad will still be good with just a couple of the above.

Next, make the dressing. In a small dish, add the remaining 1½ tbsp of olive oil, lemon juice, Dijon mustard, balsamic vinegar, and lemon peel. Mix well, then add to the salad. Toss well, then transfer the salad to serving plates.

Once the squash is done, allow it to cool for 5 minutes. Top the salad with the squash, then scatter 1 tbsp of pine nuts over each serving.

Almond Chicken

Here is a topping for chicken, but it is excellent over fish and pork as well.

- 4 oz almonds
- 2 tbsp olive oil
- 1 cup chopped onion
- ⅔ cup chopped celery
- ½ cup chopped mushrooms
- 1 (5 oz) can water chestnuts
- 2 tbsp tamari soy sauce (wheat free!)
- sea salt and fresh ground pepper to taste
- ½ cup of chicken broth, or ½ cup water + 1 tube of Trader Joe's chicken broth concentrate

Sauté the almonds in the olive oil, using a saucepan over medium heat. Once the almonds begin to brown slightly, remove them from the pan and set them aside.

Next, add the onion and celery, then sauté until soft. Add the mushrooms, cooking for 3 minutes longer. Return the almonds, then add all of the remaining ingredients. Mix well, cook until hot. Serve over shredded chicken, or other meat of your choice.

Squash and Pepper Hash

This is great at breakfast time, or anytime!

You can use many different seasoning options with this recipe to suit your tastes.

- 1 small acorn squash (about 4 cups cubed)
- 1⅓ cups chopped onion
- 2 sweet chocolate peppers or pasilla peppers
- 2 tbsp olive oil
- sea salt and pepper to taste

Peel, halve, and seed the squash. (I usually don't bother with peeling the squash, but you can if you like.) Chop the onion. Seed, stem, and chop the peppers.

Heat the olive oil in a large skillet over medium heat. (You can adjust the oil to meet your fat block needs.) Add the squash, onion, and peppers. Sauté, turning often, for around 20 minutes. Season with sea salt and fresh ground pepper.

Paleo Pizza

I am sure that I am not alone in my occasional longing for pizza since switching to eating Paleo. Pizza is a food that seems off-limits for those following a Paleo eating plan. After all, what would pizza be without the doughy crust and cheese? I decided to try to come up with a version that would nix the grain and dairy, and still taste good! This is my basic pizza recipe. You can alter it and add whatever veggies and meats that you like to make your favorite style of pizza.

- 1 cup ground almonds or other nuts
- 3 tbsp cashew butter
- ⅓ cup egg whites
- 3 tsp olive oil, divided
- 1 large Italian sausage, cut in ½-inch slices
- 2 cloves minced garlic
- ½ cup chopped onion
- 1 chopped red pepper
- ½ cup marinara sauce
- ½ tsp oregano
- ½ tsp fennel seed
- ½ cup halved grape tomatoes

Mix ground nuts, cashew butter, and egg whites in a small bowl. Grease a pizza baking sheet or similar with 2 tsp of olive oil, then spread the "dough" mixture over it, making a ¼-inch-thick crust. Preheat the oven to 250 degrees. In a skillet, add the remaining olive oil and the sliced sausage. Cook until browned, then remove the sausage to a small bowl. Add the garlic, onions, and red pepper to the skillet. Sauté the veggies lightly, making sure not to let them get too soft.

Cover the dough with the marinara sauce, then add the meat and vegetables, excluding the tomatoes. Add the oregano and fennel seed, then bake for 30 minutes. Remove from oven, add the halved tomatoes, and serve! Use a large spatula to carefully remove the slices from the pan, as the nutty "dough" won't be as crisp as traditional grain dough. Makes 4 servings.

Egg Torte

Here is a light breakfast meal. It is traditionally made with rice, but we'll use cauliflower instead. This recipe is for one torte; make multiple tortes one at a time.

- ½ tbsp olive oil
- ¼ cup finely chopped cauliflower
- ¼ cup chopped red bell pepper
- ¼ cup chopped onion
- 1 tsp chopped serrano pepper
- 2 egg whites
- sea salt and pepper to taste
- ¼ cup fresh chopped cilantro

Place a small skillet over medium heat, adding the olive oil. Sauté the cauliflower for 2–3 minutes. Add the red pepper, onion, and serrano pepper. Sauté until the veggies are soft.

Meanwhile, whisk the two egg whites in a bowl until fluffy. Add the sautéed veggies when done, then the salt and pepper; mix well.

Add the mixture to the skillet, frying one side, then flipping. Cook until light golden brown. Serve topped with the cilantro. Repeat the process for each torte.

Greek Scallops

- 1 lb. sea scallops
- 2 tbsp olive oil
- 1 cup chopped onion
- 1 cup sliced mushrooms
- 2 cloves minced garlic
- 1 cup chopped tomatoes
- ¼ cup chopped parsley
- 2 tbsp lemon juice
- oregano to taste
- pepper to taste
- 1 hard-boiled egg, chopped
- 2 tbsp pine nuts

In a large saucepan, heat the scallops in 1 tbsp of olive oil until opaque, around 5 minutes. Transfer the scallops and liquid to a bowl and set aside. Rinse and dry the pan.

Now, heat 1 tbsp of olive oil in the pan; this time, add the onions and sauté for 2 minutes. Add the mushrooms and sauté 3–5 minutes more, then add the minced garlic and sauté for 1 more minute. Add the tomato, chopped parsley, lemon juice, oregano, and pepper. Boil, then reduce heat and simmer 5 minutes. Stir in the scallops and liquid and bring to a boil. Serve into bowls, top with the chopped hard-boiled egg and pine nuts.

THIRTEEN

◇◇◇◇◇◇◇◇◇◇◇◇◇◇◇◇◇◇◇◇◇◇◇◇◇◇◇◇◇◇◇◇◇◇◇◇◇◇◇

Supplements

◇◇◇◇◇◇◇◇◇◇◇◇◇◇◇◇◇◇◇◇◇◇◇◇◇◇◇◇◇◇◇◇◇◇◇◇◇◇◇

I receive a lot of questions about supplements, but I find it difficult to recommend many. This is not for lack of options mind you! There are thousands of individual and combination supplements in any health food store or vitamin shack. The problem is I never figured out how to ignore facts in order to fleece people of their money.

Despite the hype and promises, most supplements fail to deliver much of anything. This is not to say there are no good supplements. I love many botanical extracts for various conditions, as well as many of the substances that exist in the gray area of nutriceutical/drug. Things like Piracetam, which improves memory and prevents many of the signs of aging.

There are in fact a great number of supplements and pharmaceuticals that have some amazing properties, but people get distracted by shiny objects and think there is a short-cut around nutrition, exercise, and lifestyle changes. If I go into detail about a ton of supplements, fewer of you will actually *do* the plan in the book because you will try to supplement your way through a crap diet, no exercise, and inadequate sleep.

If I had fewer scruples, I'd just make a Paleo Solution supplement line, promise you the moon, charge you a bundle for the crap, and re-tire to a tropical island. But I'm an idiot, and I actually want to help people. I want to see you make legitimate progress. It is unlikely that any supplement or drug will benefit you more than Paleo nutrition, a little exercise, and a good night's sleep. I know, it's not very sexy, but it's the truth.

In addition to a lack of results from most supplements, there is mounting evidence that supplements may actually be harmful. High-dose antioxidants and vitamin supplementation ("high" meaning well above physiologic norms) are remarkably unimpressive in anything besides a legitimate deficiency condition and might even be problem-atic. Why might this be? Well, remember the theme of this book. When we are exposed to things that are new to our physiology or in amounts that our physiology has never seen before, we are at higher risk of developing problems. I'm sure I can find exceptions to this, but it's a pretty solid guideline to follow. Not surprisingly, the supplements I do recommend for most people are simply absent or insufficient in a modern diet.

Vitamin D

Actually we will call it "Vitamin 34 double-D." It's *that* important.

What Is It?
Vit-D's designation as a "vitamin" is a bit misleading in that it is re-ally a prohormone (the precursor of a biologically active hormone). Also, we do not need to ingest vitamin D, as we make all we need if we get adequate sunlight on our skin. Vit-D has several metabolites, but we will only consider D2 (ergocalciferol), D3 (cholcalciferol), and the active form of the hormone/vitamin calcitrol (1,25-Dihydroxycho-lecalciferol).

What Does It Do?
Vit-D is best known for its role in calcium and phosphorous metabo-lism. A deficiency of Vit-D can cause rickets, but this lowly vitamin does so much more. Vit-D is critical in:

- Fat metabolism
- Cancer prevention (cell growth and apoptosis)
- Autoimmunity (regulating and normalizing immune response)
- Fertility
- Insulin resistance
- Types 1 and 2 diabetes
- Cardiovascular disease
- Anti-inflammatory as a Cox2 inhibitor

You might find it surprising that lowly vitamin D would be my first pick as the most important supplement (it was a tight race between Vit-D and fish oil), but here is my reasoning: From a Paleolithic perspective, we are interested in controlling nutrition and lifestyle factors to bring your physiology back in line with that of our genetically identical Paleolithic ancestors. Most of these efforts will involve actions that reduce systemic inflammation. Vit-D reduces and controls inflammation from a variety of angles, and it can be tough to get enough because we generally live indoors, thus limiting our light exposure. By contrast, people who choose grass-fed meat and wild-caught fish will often get enough n-3 fats (EPA/DHA), effectively removing the need for supplemental fish oil. These folks are eating a 1:1 or a 1:2 ratio of n-3 to n-6 and are fine on that count.

Where Do We Get It?
Historically we obtained Vit-D via a photosynthetic process in which UVB radiation in sunlight converts cholesterol into D3. We can obtain Vit-D from certain animal products, such as liver or fortified dairy products, but liver offers several problems, including very high levels of Vit-A. Although Vit-A works synergistically with D, too much dietary Vit-A can act as an inhibitor of Vit-D. Interestingly, our main source of Vit-A has historically been the conversion of carotenoids (most people have heard of beta-carotene) into Vit-A (retinyl palmitate).

How Much Do We Need?
Not surprisingly, governmental recommendations for Vit-D are weaker than a simultaneous case of rickets, scurvy, and anemia! Most guidelines recommend approximately 200 IU of Vit-D (remember this is

D3), with the primary focus being placed on preventing undue bone demineralization. Virtually no thought is put toward the levels our species evolved with. Although Vit-D conversion is variable based on many factors, including skin pigmentation (darker skin makes less Vit-D relative to lighter-skinned populations), latitude (we receive more UVB at the equator and thus can potentially make more Vit-D), and air pollution (high levels of air pollution decreases UVB and thus Vit-D production), a conservative estimate places our ancestral norms at 10,000–20,000 IU of Vit-D per day due to sun exposure!

Let's look at some interesting information. Governmental recommendations for tissue and blood vitamin D levels range from ~30–35 ng/dl, whereas populations that live equatorially and receive significant sun exposure have tissue levels as high as ~65–80 ng/dl. Many studies have indicated levels above 50 ng/dl to be protective against cancer and autoimmunity, which should not be surprising, as this is likely reflective of levels normal to our Paleolithic genetics. Given the ever-growing number of benefits derived from maintaining an ancestral level of Vit-D, I think it's reasonable for most people to supplement with 2,000–5,000 IU per day of gel-cap Vit-D3. A six-month supply will likely set you back less than $10. Take this in the AM with a meal containing fat. If you would like to track blood work, you should look for a supplementation schedule that gives you ~50–65 ng/dl. Yes, this is a good bit higher than the government recommended levels, but I think the benefits easily outweigh any potential downsides. Folks who suffer from hyperparathyroid disease will need to maintain dosages less than 1,000 IU/day, as they are at increased risk of Vit-D toxicity.

Sun Exposure

In their outstanding book *Protein Power: Life Plan*, Doctors Michael and Mary Eades recommend sunbathing as a means of supplementing Vit-D. They recommend a schedule based on latitude and your natural level of skin pigmentation to gauge how much sun you need to produce adequate Vit-D. This is actually my preferred method for you to reach your Vit-D quota, but in all honesty, this is *very* hard for most folks to do. The key to this whole process is "safe, reasonable increases in sun exposure." That is hard as hell to do if you live in a relatively cold/

overcast environment, have kids, or your job does not allow you to hang out in the sun for twenty to sixty minutes per day.

All this considered, if you can construct a lifestyle that allows you to incrementally increase your sun exposure so that you can reach desired levels of Vit-D, go for it. If you are concerned about skin cancer because of this sun exposure, keep in mind, safe, incremental sun exposure (not burning your skin) *decreases* your likelihood of developing a host of cancers far more than it increases your likelihood of developing skin cancer. The main risk factor in skin cancer appears to be infrequent, severe burns. Use your head—if you can't help but scorch yourself because you drink too many NorCal margaritas when you are in the sun, just stick with Vit-D supplements. If you want to play with sunbathing to make your Vit-D, you will find resources on the Robbwolf.com website to help you calculate your UV exposure for a given area.

HINI and Vit-D

Although most of the conditions related to Vit-D deficiency are chronic, degenerative diseases, Vit-D's power is perhaps best illustrated in the case of acute, infectious disease such as the H1N1 influenza virus. H1N1 has received massive media attention in the past few years due to deaths and significant illness caused by the H1N1 variant. The ultimate fear is that a form of influenza that killed millions of people worldwide in 1918 will reemerge. And, something like it eventually will.

What we have learned from the H1N1 epidemiology is low Vit-D is not only a risk factor for contracting the disease, it is also a factor in how severely the disease manifests in a given individual. Yet again, levels above 50 ng/dl appear to decrease the likelihood of contracting the virus or of suffering the "cytokine storm" that appears to be the mechanism behind deaths caused by the virus. Not surprisingly, any factors contributing to inflammation appear to worsen the cytokine storm.

Omega-3 Fats

I went into significant detail about n-3 fats in chapter 5, so no need to rehash that here. Keep in mind, we are concerned about two things with regards to n-3 fats: type and ratio. The type we want are the long-chain forms (EPA and DHA) found primarily in wild fish and grass-fed meat. The ratio we are shooting for is 1:1 to 1:2 n-3 to n-6.

What Does It Do?

If you recall from chapter 5, what *doesn't* it do?! Interestingly, we see multiple disease conditions affected by our n-3 status. N-3s affect a host of critical hormonal and cell-to-cell communication systems including prostaglandins, leukotriens, cytokines, and thromboxanes. This means n-3 fats have influence on:

- Cancer (cell differentiation and apoptosis)
- Autoimmunity (regulating and normalizing immune response)
- Insulin sensitivity/resistance
- Neurodegeneration
- Recovery from activity
- Fertility

Where Do We Get It?

As I mentioned before, we historically obtained our essential fats, both n-3 and n-6, from dietary sources of wild game, seafood, and less appetizing sources like grubs and insects. Our modern, grain-fed food supply, complete with refined vegetable oils rich in n-6, has completely altered the critical balance of n-3/n-6 in our modern diet.

How Much Do We Need?

How much fish oil we need is highly subjective. For individuals who show signs of systemic inflammation, are overweight, or have been diagnosed with a condition related to insulin resistance or autoimmunity, the dosage may be quite high initially. As much as one gram of EPA/DHA for every ten pounds of body weight per day. That means total EPA/DHA! Your product will vary in how much it contains. You

1g/10 lbs of Body Weight	
150 lbs	15 g
200 lbs	20 g
250 lbs	25 g
300 lbs	30 g

Fish oil recommendations for sick, overweight, and highly inflamed individuals.

.25g/10 lbs of Body Weight	
150 lbs	3.75 g
200 lbs	5 g
250 lbs	6.25 g
300 lbs	7.5 g

Fish oil recommendations for lean, athletic individuals.

can use the online calculator made by our friends at Whole9life.com/fish-oil/

This may seem like a lot, but you will only stay at this level for a month or two to accelerate the healing process.

If you are generally healthy and athletic and eating well (lean conventional sources of meat), you are fine with a dosage between .25 and .5 g/10 lbs body weight. If you are getting the bulk of your protein from grass-fed and wild-caught sources, and you are not taking in large amounts of n-6 heavy fats (sunflower seeds, soy bean oil, etc.), then you may not need to supplement at all. How will you know how much you need? You can do a simple EPA blood test and get a general idea as to your status but, honestly, I've had few situations where that test was necessary. A simpler approach is to just go by how you feel. If you have reversed insulin resistance, lost weight, and are looking and feeling great, your need for fish oil will have decreased. Most of our healthy, active clients supplement at .25 g/10 lbs body weight (see table above).

Brands and Varieties

There are hundreds of fish oil suppliers. Some are great, some not so great. Quality varies significantly, but I really like the following companies:

Nordic Naturals
Carlsons
Barleans

Capsule or Liquid?

Well, that depends. It's easier to get a large amount of fish oil down in liquid form. Many people complain of the need to take a handful of capsules with each meal. Keep in mind, this is a vital nutrient that *should* be in our food supply, but is not. The people who balk at the amount of fish oil they need to take seem to be the same people who have problems losing weight, turning around their health conditions, and making progress. Give this stuff a shot for a month or two and you will be amazed by the progress you make.

Should You Get the "Pharmaceutical Grade Fish Oil"?

Ultra-purified fish oil is more expensive, but you get what you pay for. Many people who have GI problems with standard fish oil have no such problems with ultra-purified fish oil.

What about Contaminants Like Mercury and PCBs?

Mercury is a highly toxic metal that, unfortunately, accumulates in many varieties of seafood. Inorganic mercury is transformed into methyl-mercury, and this compound can find its way into the food web. Larger, longer-lived critters tend to accumulate more mercury than smaller, shorter-lived species. Mercury's toxicity stems from its effects on nerves and critical enzyme systems. Mercury is bad, and overconsumption of mercury is a real issue in certain situations, but fish oil is *not* a source of mercury intake. You see, mercury binds tightly to proteins, and fish oil, even relatively unprocessed fish oil, has virtually no protein and, therefore, no mercury.

PCBs are organic contaminants from manufacturing, agriculture, and plastics. PCBs can and do accumulate in the fatty portions of fish but, again, smaller varieties of fish contain significantly lower levels. Sardines and mackerel are thus good sources for your fish oil. This is also an argument to use the ultrapurified varieties, as virtually all contaminants are removed in the micro-distillation process.

What about the EPA/DHA Ratio?

This will vary based on the source for the fish oil. In general, an equal ratio is a good option, although some research indicates a DHA-heavy formulation is better for reasons of improved neurological function.

What about Moms and Kids?

Pregnant or breastfeeding moms should focus on a DHA-heavy product. DHA is the main constituent needed by growing brains, be they fetal or toddler. Children below the age of three should *only* be given supplements with DHA, as too much EPA can limit arachidonic acid production in children and thus stunt neurological development. Dosage for kids, according to the DHA-EPA-Omega-3 institute, should be: 0.5 g for infants, 0.7 g for kids ages one to three years old, stepping up to 1–2 g per day for kids ages four to thirteen.

DHA from Algae

One product may solve many of the above issues, while also addressing concerns of over fishing and sustainability.

DHA derived from algae is not only perfect for moms and kids, but it is also free of contaminants, is sustainable, and should become less expensive as demand grows for this product. Conveniently, DHA converts to EPA in our bodies, so this supplement is truly a good option.

Magnesium

Magnesium is a vital mineral that unfortunately takes a backseat to its divalent cousin, calcium. Interestingly, we hear about calcium all the time, but rarely do we hear about magnesium, which played a large role in the evolution of our genetics. Magnesium comes in several varieties, including magnesium oxide, magnesium chelates, and magnesium citrate, just to name a few of the more popular options. Your best option for a supplement is the magnesium citrate form, as it appears to be the best absorbed.

What Does It Do?

In addition to being critical in a dizzying number of enzymatic reactions in our bodies, magnesium has influence in blood clotting, energy production, muscle contraction, and nerve transmission. Magnesium deficiency appears to be a player in:

- Insulin resistance
- Cardiovascular disease

- Chronic fatigue/fibromyalgia
- High blood pressure

Where Do We Get It?
Fruits and vegetables, particularly dark green vegetables, have historically been our best sources for magnesium.

How Much Do We Need?
Although the recommended daily allowance for magnesium is 300–400 mg per day for adults, this is a paltry amount as compared to a simple reconstruction of our ancestral diet using commonly available modern foods. More realistic numbers are in the 1,200–2,000 mg (1.2–2 g) per day range. Our modern diet's heavy reliance on dairy products and grains have displaced fruits and vegetables, generally increasing calcium intake, while our intake of magnesium has fallen to levels well below that seen in our ancestral past. Interestingly, however, our bones have paid the price. Although our intake of calcium is relatively high, magnesium is a critical cofactor in bone formation and actually increases calcium absorption. Instead of focusing on more calcium to improve bone density, we should focus on weight-bearing exercise, adequate Vit-D levels, a diet devoid of antinutrients and gut irritants, and ancestral levels of magnesium.

I have seen a number of people benefit from supplemental magnesium (myself included), and the most effective form I have seen are varieties of "fizzy" magnesium drinks such as Natural Calm. Magnesium can be very relaxing, almost sedating for many people. 400–600 mg of magnesium citrate mixed in warm water before bed is so relaxing I actually look forward to it. If you are the rare person who is a "paradoxical responder" and magnesium stimulates you, just take it in the AM upon waking.

Can You Take Too Much Magnesium?
Yes, but the results are not too dire unless you find yourself trapped away from a privy. Magnesium can be a potent laxative!

Digestive Aides

Digestive aides were not in the ancestral diet, of course, but they may be of benefit to great many people who suffer from low stomach acid and weak digestion. The digestive aids I recommend contain betaine-hydrochloride, ox bile, proteases, lipases, and amylases.

What Does It Do?

Betaine-HCL helps to increase stomach acid. Although only a limited amount of digestion occurs in the stomach, much of the signaling that occurs later in the digestive process is initiated by a high concentration of stomach acid. Many people are wary of high stomach acid due to gastric reflux, but the vast majority of these problems are an outgrowth of high insulin levels and grain intolerance.

Ox bile helps to emulsify fats, making them more available for digestion. *Remember*, that means essential fats, antioxidants, and fat-soluble vitamins! You *do* want good fat digestion and absorption.

Proteases, Lipases, and Amylases

These are digestive enzymes normally released by the pancreas, and they digest protein, fats, and carbohydrates respectively. Low stomach acid or inflammation to the pancreas caused by grain intolerance, abnormal gut flora, or high insulin levels can decrease the amount of digestive enzymes released into the small intestines, thus reducing the effectiveness of our digestion.

Where Do We Get It?

Supplement only! There are a number of products like this on the market, but I really like the NowFoods: Super Enzymes product. It is inexpensive and very effective.

How Much Do We Need?

Digestive support is particularly important if you have suffered GI problems in the past, have an autoimmune disease, or significant systemic inflammation. Folks who have had their gall bladders removed really *need* to follow a protocol like this one:

For folks using a digestive aid with betaine-HCL, start with one capsule per meal for a day or two. Do you feel any type of "warmth" in the epigastric region (at the bottom of your breast bone where the ribs meet)? If so, you may not need digestive support. If you do not feel warmth, take two caps with each meal for a day or two. Warmth? Keep following this progress until you are up to five caps per meal. If you are *still* not feeling warmth, just hang at this dosage until you do start to feel warmth after a meal. Whatever your dosage, when you start to feel warmth, dial your dosage down by one cap per meal until you are digesting your food without supplemental enzymes.

Do I Use These Digestive Enzymes If I Am Eating a Fruit Bowl?

No! Remember, the majority of your meals need to be made of protein, veggies, and fat. The main things the enzymes are helping you break down are protein and fat. If you eat a meal without protein and fat, you are wasting your efforts.

How Long Will I Need to Use Digestive Enzymes?

I don't know; it all depends on how weak your digestion is, your stress level, and how compliant you are with the food, exercise, and life-style recommendations. I was pretty sick after my "adventures in vegan land," and it took me several years to really get my digestion put back together. I then chose to start a business, skimp on my sleep, and travel constantly for work, with the result being adrenal fatigue and blown digestion. *Again.* Be smarter than me, please!

Probiotics

The term *probiotics* refers to a broad and ever-expanding group of microorganisms that inhabit the intestines and are absolutely critical to the normal functioning of our digestion and immune system. Bacterial strains include various *Lactobacili*, *bifidum*, and *bacilli species*, but there are also beneficial fungi such as *Saccharomyces boulardi*.

What Does It Do?

I could write a book on probiotics alone, and the title would be amazing: *Bacteria, Poop, and You: How Beneficial Bacteria Can Make You Healthier and Look Great in a Bikini.* Seriously though, probiotics are massively underrated and are just now receiving the research focus they deserve. The roles these bacteria play are varied, but they are critical in not only the digestive process, but also in actually protecting the gut lining. Our beneficial flora (the living mass of bacteria in our intestines) actually line the villi and microvilli in such a tight association that the bacteria are literally the first layer of our intestines. These bacteria displace potentially pathogenic bacteria, yeast, and parasites; help us to digest macronutrients; and are responsible for the production of various vitamins from precursor molecules. We are also discovering that our gut flora has tight communication and influence with both our immune and nervous systems. Certain types of mouth bacteria have even been shown to be helpful in preventing periodontal disease. For being kept in the dark and only allowed to associate with poo, these little buggers do a lot!

Where Do We Get It?

Most people are familiar with various fermented foods such as yogurt, kefir, miso, kimchi, and raw sauerkraut. All of these foods (if not pasteurized) provide live cultures of beneficial bacteria. Those of you with a queasy stomach should just skip this next part! Where did we obtain our beneficial flora in the past, before fermented foods such as yogurt and kimchi? Well, our ancestors were particularly fond of the intestinal contents of herbivores. I know, it's not the greatest thing to imagine, but similar bacteria inhabit herbivore GI tracts, and this was likely a large and consistent source of beneficial bacteria.

How Much Do We Need?

There are no specific guidelines or RDA for probiotics, but I think it's important to supplement frequently with a broad range of sources. Fermented foods are certainly an option and, as you might have guessed, I'd recommend focusing on fermented vegetables such as sauerkrauts, kimchi, and similar foods. You can find live, unpasteurized versions of these foods at most hippy super markets, but if you are industrious, you can make them yourself at home. Keep in mind, most of these foods are quite high in salt, and this can be problematic for some people with high blood pressure or sleep problems. You can also of course make use of fermented dairy products, but these carry the same problems of all dairy: elevated insulin levels and potential gut irritation.

If you are using foods as your main source, try to get a serving or two of probiotic-rich foods daily. If the food route seems like a hassle or you just want to make sure you have covered all your bases, you can use a mixed probiotic such as Jarro-Dophilus or products from New Chapter. Take these supplements on an empty stomach first thing in the morning, and just follow the label recommendations. Remember, those are live cultures! Use them in a timely manner and keep them in the refrigerator.

Saccharomyces boulardi

If you should find yourself in the unfortunate situation of taking antibiotics, I highly recommend you take the beneficial yeast, *S. boulardi* (SB). Antibiotics tend to not only take out pathogenic bacteria, but also our beneficial flora. This can set us up for yeast infections from nasty critters like *Candida albicans* or bacteria such as *Helicobacter pylori*. Since SB is a yeast, it is unaffected by antibiotics. SB also makes a nice addition to your travel bag as it is heat stable. Start taking SB five to seven days prior to travel and while on the road, and you can decrease your likelihood of succumbing to traveler's diarrhea.

Iodine

Iodine is a trace element that might be lacking in a modern interpretation of a Paleolithic diet.

What Does It Do?
Iodine is a key constituent in thyroid hormones thyroxine (T4) and triiodothyronine (T3). T3 is the more biologically active of the hormones and is critical in energy management, fertility, hormone regulation, and a number of other vital processes.

Where Do We Get It?

Kelp, seaweed, and seafood are excellent sources of iodine. Unless you live in an area where the soil is rich in iodine (few place are), you will likely need some kind of supplemental iodine or make a concerted effort to include some seaweed or kelp in your program. Iodized table salt has been a common and convenient source of iodine for many people, but with the adoption of Paleo eating, most people find their salt intake to decrease markedly.

How Much Do We Need?

A safe dose for most people is 150 micrograms/day, although women who are pregnant or lactating may need as much as 200–300 micrograms per day. On the topic of women, I have noticed a number of females who were suffering from signs and symptoms of hyperinsulinism, including amenorrhea, or reproductive difficulties. These women adopted a Paleo diet, started exercising, and slept better, but did not see improvements in their estrogen/insulin-related issues as much as I'd like to see. Iodine is quite important in estrogen metabolism, so I recommended that these women add in 150 mcg of iodine per day and they saw almost immediate improvement in their symptoms.

I really like seaweed, as commonly found in Japanese food, but it's tough to know how much iodine you obtain from these sources. If you suspect an iodine deficiency, I'd suggest blood work to check your thyroid levels and supplementing with 150 mcg/day. Many people who register in the "low but normal" range for thyroid hormone notice significant improvements in how they feel, in cold tolerance, and other issues related to proper thyroid function when they increase their intake of iodine. Average values are just that—averages of a vast number of people. That number may not be what is optimal for you, however.

R-alpha Lipoic Acid + N-acetyl-L carnitine

This is a combo recommendation and it deviates a bit from the other items in that it's really something for "optimizing" things like cognition and sexual function. Alpha lipoic acid (ALA) is a potent fat- and water-soluble antioxidant. N-acetyl-L-carnitine (NAC) is a modified form of carnitine, which is an important amino acid.

What Does It Do?

ALA is not only a fat- and water-soluble antioxidant, but it also helps to restore the antioxidant activities of vitamins C and E. ALA is also helpful for reversing insulin resistance and is particularly helpful for diabetic neuropathy. NAC has been shown to help reverse the signs and symptoms of aging and dementia. In addition to this, NAC is important in fat metabolism, as carnitine acts as a carrier molecule for fats entering the mitochondria of cells to be used for energy.

Where Do We Get It?

(ALA) is found in large amounts in grass-fed or wild meats. Grain-fed meat unfortunately has virtually no ALA. NAC is made in the body from carnitine.

There are many companies such as Jarrow that offer a combination of NAC and ALA in one capsule or tablet, but you can also buy these items individually to dial in your dosage.

How Much Do We Need?

You will need to play with this a little to find your optimum dosage, but 600– 1,200 mg of NAC taken with 1,000–2,000 mg of ALA first thing in the morning on an empty stomach has a remarkable ability to "clear the fog." It is not stimulating in the way caffeine is, but it really cranks up the wattage between the ears! You will find this helpful on most mornings, but particularly so on those days after you've had a few too many NorCal margaritas! Some of you may find the ALA drops your blood sugar too much unless you take it with a little food. Just be aware that ALA *does* improve insulin sensitivity, and this can mean a decrease in blood sugar past what is comfortable.

Epilogue

WOW! So, that was a lot. How ya doing? Need a hug? I hope that you give this a shot. Take 30 days, commit to the program, then re-evaluate. It is completely reasonable to ask the question "Is it worth it to do this?" Does the cost-benefit analysis play out in favor of a Paleo Solution for your life? Of the thousands of people I've worked with the answer is an emphatic "yes, it's worth it". Most folks tackle this as a "diet" initially, but it morphs into a viable, long term lifestyle. People have different levels of buy-in and that's great. The ideas are here to make your life better, not shackle you to an uptight ideology.

So, where do you go from here? Well, community and support are critical to all of our successes, so I'd suggest you come and hang out at www.robbwolf.com. You will find quite a number of resources and portals to other folks who are knowledgeable about this Paleo/Primal life-way. I have links to many fantastic blogs and websites, but a few need attention here. My mentor, Prof. Loren Cordain, has an amazing site at www.thepaleodiet.com. If you look in my reference section, you will find much of his work cited therein. Make sure to read his book, *The Paleo Diet,* and for the endurance athletes amongst you, *The Paleo Diet For Athletes.* If you are looking for gear to outfit a home gym, I recommend you check out www.cathletics.com. For gymnastics rings (for body-rows and many other movements), plus a gymnastics oriented workout, see Coach Christopher Sommer's http://gymnasticbodies.com. If you need a simple, effective daily workout to follow there is nothing that can compare to Coach Michael Rutherfords' program: www.coachrut.blogspot.com. Another great resource for training and Primal movement is www.movnat.com.

One area that people struggle with is finding Paleo friendly snacks and quick meals. A fantastic solution is Paleo Brands: http://paleo-brands.com/. This includes a complete line of gourmet (gluten free, grain free, dairy free) meals built from grass-fed meat, wild caught fish, and organic vegetables. Paleo Brands also offers a line of Paleo snacks, which includes grass-fed beef jerky and delicious almond/honey Paleo cookies.

Please share your experiences with the Paleo Solution at www.robbwolf.com. It is not my intention for this to be a one-way communication. I've shared my story with you, now it's your turn to do the same.

References

Anthropology
Chapter Two: Hunter Gatherers Are Us

Ultraviolet radiation represents an evolutionary selective pressure for the south-to-north gradient of the MTHFR 677TT genotype. Cordain L, Hickey MS. Am J Clin Nutr. 2006 Nov;84(5):1243; author reply 1244-5.

The hunter-gatherer diet. Hays JH. Mayo Clin Proc. 2004 May;79(5):703; author reply 703-4, 707.

Implications of Plio-Pleistocene Hominin Diets for Modern Humans. In: Early Hominin Diets: The Known, the Unknown, and the Unknowable. Cordain L.,Ungar, P (Ed.), Oxford University Press, Oxford, 2006, pp 363-83.

Evolutionary health promotion. Eaton SB, Strassman BI, Nesse RM, Neel JV, Ewald PW, Williams GC, Weder AB, Eaton SB 3rd, Lindeberg S, Konner MJ, Mysterud I, Cordain L. Prev Med 2002; 34:109-118.

Old genes, new fuels: Nutritional changes since agriculture. Eaton, S.B., Cordain, L.World Rev Nutr Diet 1997; 81:26-37.

A brief review of the archaeological evidence for Palaeolithic and Neolithic subsistence. MP Richards1* European Journal of Clinical Nutrition (2002) 56 ß 2002 Nature Publishing Group All rights reserved 0954–3007/02.

Studying Children in "Hunter-Gatherer" Societies. Reflections from a Nayaka Perspective. Bird-David- www.vancouver.wsu.edu/fac/hewlett/Anth302/Bird-David.pdf.

Bone density in Sadlermiut Eskimo. Mazess RB. Hum Biol. 1966 Feb;38(1):42-9.

BONES OF CONTENTION THE POLITICAL ECONOMY OF HEIGHT INEQUALITY. Carles Boix and Frances Rosenbluth. www.princeton.edu/~cboix/bones.pdf.

Long Term History of the Human Diet. Glynn Li. Isac and Jeanne M. Sept. www.ltspeed.com/bjblinder/book/secure/chapter4.pdf.

Dental Health Diet and Social Status among Central African Foragers and Farmers. PHILLIP L. WALKER1,3 and BARRY S. HEWLETT 2,4. American Anthropologist, Volume 92 Issue 2, Pages 383 - 398.

Evolution in Health and Disease. Second Edition. EDITED BY Stephen C. Stearns and Jacob C. Koella. Oxford University Press. 2008-ISBN 978–0–19–920745–9.

Evolutionary explanations in medical and health profession courses: are you answering your students' "why" questions? EugeneEHarris and Avelin A Malyango. BMC Medical Education 2005, 5:16 doi:10.1186/1472-6920-5-16. Received: 22 September 2004.

The Fertility of Agricultural and Non-Agricultural Traditional Societies. GILLIAN R. BENTLEY, TONY GOLDBERG, AND GRAZYNA JASIENSKA J. Population Studies, 47 (1993), 269-281.

Milk in the island of Chole [Tanzania] is high in lauric, myristic, arachidonic and docosahexaenoic acids, and low in linoleic acid. Reconstructed diet of infants born to our ancestors living in tropical coastal regions. Remko S. Kuipersa, Ella N. Smita, Jan van der Meulenb, D.A. Janneke Dijck-Brouwera, E. Rudy Boersmac, d, Frits A.J. Muskieta. Prostaglandins, Leukotrienes and Essential Fatty Acids 76 (2007) 221–233.

Is Lamarckian evolution relevant to medicine? Adam E Handel 1,2 and Sreeram V Ramagopalan Handel and Ramagopalan. BMC Medical Genetics 2010, 11:73.

"The Worst Mistake In The History Of The Human Race" by Jared Diamond, Prof. UCLA School of Medicine. Discover-May 1987, pp. 64-66.

ANEMIA AMONG PREHISTORIC INDIANS OF THE AMERICAN SOUTHWEST. Phillip L. Walker. Health and disease in the prehistoric southwest. Charles F. Merbs and Robert J Miller, 1985. Arizona State University. Anthropological research papers NO .34.

An overview on the nutrition transition and its health implications: the Bellagio meeting. Public Health Nutrition: 5(1A), 93–103 DOI: 10.1079/PHN2001280.

Stable Isotope Analyses in Human Nutritional Ecology. HENRY P. SCHWARCZ AND MARGARET J. SCHOENINGER. YEARBOOK OF PHYSICAL ANTHROPOLOGY 34:283-321 (1991).

Evolution in health and medicine Sackler colloquium: Evolutionary perspectives on health and medicine. Stearns SC, Nesse RM, Govindaraju DR, Ellison PT. Proc Natl Acad Sci U S A. 2010 Jan 26;107 Suppl 1:1691-5.

What Ancient Human Teeth Can Reveal? Demography, Health, Nutrition and Biological Relations in Luistari Master thesis in archaeology. Kati Salo, Supervisors: prof. Ebba During (University of Stockholm), assistant Tuija Kirkinen (University of Helsinki) 2005-05-06.

The etiology and porotic hyperostosis among the prehistoric and historic Anasazi Indians of Southwestern United States. El-Najjar MY, Ryan DJ, Turner CG 2nd, Lozoff B. Am J Phys Anthropol. 1976 May;44(3):477-87.

Nutrition and health in agriculturalists and hunter-gatherers: a case study of two prehistoric populations in Nutritional Anthropology. Cassidy CM. Eds Jerome NW et al. 1980 Redgrave Publishing Company, Pleasantville, NY pg 117-145.

Insulin
Chapter Three-Five

Sarcopenic obesity and inflammation in the InCHIANTI study. Schrager MA, Metter EJ, Simonsick E, Ble A, Bandinelli S, Lauretani F, Ferrucci L. Longitudinal Studies Section, Clinical Research Branch, National Institute on Aging, National Institutes of Health, Baltimore, MD 21225, USA. J Appl Physiol. 2007 Mar;102(3):919-25. Epub 2006 Nov 9.

Insulin, Insulin-Like Growth Factors and Colon Cancer: A Review of the Evidence. Edward Giovannucci. The American Society for Nutritional Sciences J. Nutr. 131:3109S-3120S, November 2001. Supplement: AICR's 11th Annual Research Conference on Diet, Nutrition and Cancer.

Hyperinsulinemic diseases of civilization: more than just Syndrome X. Cordain L, Eades MR, Eades MD. Comp Biochem Physiol A Mol Integr Physiol. 2003 Sep;136(1):95-112.

Nutrition, insulin, insulin-like growth factors and cancer. Giovannucci E. Horm Metab Res. 2003 Nov-Dec;35(11-12):694-704.

Hypoglycemia and resistance to ketoacidosis in a subject without functional insulin receptors. Ogilvy-Stuart AL, Soos MA, Hands SJ, Anthony MY, Dunger DB, O'Rahilly S. J Clin Endocrinol Metab. 2001 Jul;86(7):3319-26.

Is there a role for a low-carbohydrate ketogenic diet in the management of prostate cancer? Mavropoulos JC, Isaacs WB, Pizzo SV, Freedland SJ. Urology. 2006 Jul;68(1):15-8.

The Ancestral Biomedical Environment In: Endothelial Biomedicine. Eaton SB, Cordain L, Sebastian A. W.C. Aird (Ed), Cambridge University Press, 2007, pp. 129-134.

Anticonvulsant mechanisms of the ketogenic diet. Bough KJ, Rho JM. Epilepsia. 2007 Jan;48(1):43-58.

Rho Kinases in Cardiovascular Physiology and Pathophysiology. Gervaise Loirand, Patrice Guérin, Pierre Pacaud. Circulation Research. 2006;98:322.

Gene-diet interactions in brain aging and neurodegenerative disorders. Mattson MP. Ann Intern Med. 2003 Sep 2;139(5 Pt 2):441-4.

An evolutionary analysis of the etiology and pathogenesis of juvenile-onset myopia. Cordain L, Eaton SB, Brand Miller J, Lindeberg S, Jensen C. Acta Ophthalmologica Scandinavica, 2002; 80:125-135.

Genotype, obesity and cardiovascular disease--has technical and social advancement outstripped evolution? Zimmet P, Thomas CR. J Intern Med. 2003 Aug;254(2):114-25.

Coronary endothelial dysfunction in the insulin-resistant state is linked to abnormal pteridine metabolism and vascular oxidative stress. Shinozaki K, Hirayama A, Nishio Y, Yoshida Y, Ohtani T, Okamura T, Masada M, Kikkawa R,Kodama K, Kashiwagi A. J Am Coll Cardiol. 2001 Dec;38(7):1821-8.

Evolution, body composition, insulin receptor competition, and insulin resistance. Eaton SB, Cordain L, Sparling PB. Prev Med. 2009;49:283-85.

Syndrome X: Just the tip of the hyperinsulinemia iceberg. Cordain L. Medikament 2001; 6:46-51.

Insulin regulation of gene expression and concentrations of white adipose tissue-derived proteins in vivo in healthy men: relation to adiponutrin. Faraj M, Beauregard G, Loizon E, Moldes M, Clément K, Tahiri Y, Cianflone K, Vidal H, Rabasa-Lhoret R. J Endocrinol. 2006 Nov;191(2):427-35.

Insulin: understanding its action in health and disease. Sonksen P, Sonksen J. Br J Anaesth. 2000 Jul;85(1):69-79.

Insulin resistance in rheumatoid arthritis: the impact of the anti-TNF-alpha therapy. Gonzalez-Gay MA, Gonzalez-Juanatey C, Vazquez-Rodriguez TR, Miranda-Filloy JA, Llorca J. Ann N Y Acad Sci. 2010 Apr;1193(1):153-9.

Role of insulin, insulin-like growth factor-1, hyperglycaemic food and milk consumption in the pathogenesis of acne vulgaris. Melnik BC, Schmitz G. Exp Dermatol. 2009 Oct;18(10):833-41. Epub 2009 Aug 25.

Addison's disease and the regulation of potassium: the role of insulin and aldosterone. Harvey TC. Med Hypotheses. 2007;69(5):1120-6. Epub 2007 Apr 24.

Insulin resistance predicts mortality in nondiabetic individuals in the U.S. Ausk KJ, Boyko EJ, Ioannou GN. Diabetes Care. 2010 Jun;33(6):1179-85. Epub 2010 Mar 3.

Insulin sensitivity in patients with primary aldosteronism: a follow-up study. Catena C, Lapenna R, Baroselli S, Nadalini E, Colussi G, Novello M, Favret G, Melis A, Cavarape A, Sechi LA. J Clin Endocrinol Metab. 2006 Sep;91(9):3457-63. Epub 2006 Jul 5.

Kynurenines in chronic neurodegenerative disorders: future therapeutic strategies. Zádori D, Klivényi P, Vámos E, Fülöp F, Toldi J, Vécsei L. J Neural Transm. 2009 Nov;116(11):1403-9. Epub 2009 Jul 18.

Inflammation, depression and dementia: are they connected? Leonard BE. Neurochem Res. 2007 Oct;32(10):1749-56. Epub 2007 Aug 20.

Gluttony, sloth and the metabolic syndrome: a roadmap to lipotoxicity. Unger RH, Scherer PE. Trends Endocrinol Metab. 2010 Jun;21(6):345-52. Epub 2010 Mar 10.

Manipulation of brain kynurenines: glial targets, neuronal effects, and clinical opportunities. Schwarcz R, Pellicciari R. J Pharmacol Exp Ther. 2002 Oct;303(1):1-10.

Methionine residue 35 is important in amyloid beta-peptide-associated free radical oxidative stress. Varadarajan S, Yatin S, Kanski J, Jahanshahi F, Butterfield DA. Brain Res Bull. 1999 Sep 15;50(2):133-41.

Methionine oxidation by reactive oxygen species: reaction mechanisms and relevance to Alzheimer's disease. Schöneich C. Biochim Biophys Acta. 2005 Jan 17;1703(2):111-9. Epub 2004 Oct 27.

Methionine residue 35 is critical for the oxidative stress and neurotoxic properties of Alzheimer's amyloid beta-peptide 1-42. Butterfield DA, Kanski J. Peptides. 2002 Jul;23(7):1299-309.

Role of nuclear receptors in the modulation of insulin secretion in lipid-induced insulin resistance. Sugden MC, Holness MJ. Biochem Soc Trans. 2008 Oct;36(Pt 5):891-900.

Hypothalamic orexin stimulates feeding-associated glucose utilization in skeletal muscle via sympathetic nervous system. Shiuchi T, Haque MS, Okamoto S, Inoue T, Kageyama H, Lee S, Toda C, Suzuki A, Bachman ES,Kim YB, Sakurai T, Yanagisawa M, Shioda S, Imoto K, Minokoshi Y. Cell Metab. 2009 Dec;10(6):466-80.

MyD88 signaling in the CNS is required for development of fatty acid-induced leptin resistance and diet-induced obesity. Kleinridders A, Schenten D, Könner AC, Belgardt BF, Mauer J, Okamura T, Wunderlich FT,Medzhitov R, Brüning JC. Cell Metab. 2009 Oct;10(4):249-59.

Permanent impairment of insulin resistance from pregnancy to adulthood: the primary basic risk factor of chronic Western diseases. Melnik BC. Med Hypotheses. 2009 Nov;73(5):670-81. Epub 2009 Jun 9.

Cholesterol lowering, cardiovascular diseases, and the rosuvastatin-JUPITER controversy: a critical reappraisal. de Lorgeril M, Salen P, Abramson J, Dodin S, Hamazaki T, Kostucki W, Okuyama H, Pavy B, Rabaeus M. Arch Intern Med. 2010 Jun 28;170(12):1032-6.

Nutrient overload, insulin resistance, and ribosomal protein S6 kinase 1, S6K1. Um SH, D'Alessio D, Thomas G. Cell Metab. 2006 Jun;3(6):393-402.

Targeting energy metabolism in brain cancer: review and hypothesis. Seyfried TN, Mukherjee P. Nutr Metab (Lond). 2005 Oct 21;2:30.

The thrifty epigenotype: an acquired and heritable predisposition for obesity and diabetes? Stöger R. Bioessays. 2008 Feb;30(2):156-66.

The immunomodulatory effects of estrogens: clinical relevance in immune-mediated rheumatic diseases. Cutolo M, Brizzolara R, Atzeni F, Capellino S, Straub RH, Puttini PC. Ann N Y Acad Sci. 2010 Apr;1193(1):36-42.

Triglycerides induce leptin resistance at the blood-brain barrier. Banks WA, Coon AB, Robinson SM, Moinuddin A, Shultz JM, Nakaoke R, Morley JE. Diabetes. 2004 May;53(5):1253-60.

Evolution, body composition, insulin receptor competition, and insulin resistance. Eaton SB, Cordain L, Sparling PB. Prev Med. 2009 Oct;49(4):283-5. Epub 2009 Aug 15.

Molecular identification of a danger signal that alerts the immune system to dying cells. Shi Y, Evans JE, Rock KL. Nature. 2003 Oct 2;425(6957):516-21. Epub 2003 Sep 7.

Antidiabetic effects of IGFBP2, a leptin-regulated gene. Hedbacker K, Birsoy K, Wysocki RW, Asilmaz E, Ahima RS, Farooqi IS, Friedman JM Cell Metab. 2010 Jan;11(1):11-22.

Attenuation of insulin secretion by insulin-like growth factor 1 is mediated through activation of phosphodiesterase 3B. Allan Z. Zhao,* Hong Zhao,* Jeanette Teague,† Wilfred Fujimoto,† and Joseph A. Beavo*‡ Proc Natl Acad Sci U S A. 1997 April 1; 94(7): 3223–3228.

High-insulinogenic nutrition--an etiologic factor for obesity and the metabolic syndrome? Kopp W. Metabolism. 2003 Jul;52(7):840-4. Am J Clin Nutr. 2008 Nov;88(5):1189-90. How safe is fructose for persons with or without diabetes? Sánchez-Lozada LG, Le M, Segal M, Johnson RJ.

High-fructose corn syrup causes characteristics of obesity in rats: Increased body weight, body fat and triglyceride levels. Bocarsly ME, Powell ES, Avena NM, Hoebel BG. Pharmacol Biochem Behav. 2010 Feb 26. [Epub ahead of print]

Mechanism of ATP-binding cassette transporter A1-mediated cellular lipid efflux to apolipoprotein A-I and formation of high density lipoprotein particles. Vedhachalam C, Duong PT, Nickel M, Nguyen D, Dhanasekaran P, Saito H, Rothblat GH, Lund-Katz S, Phillips MC. J Biol Chem. 2007 Aug 24;282(34):25123-30. Epub 2007 Jun 29.

Does chronic glycolysis accelerate aging? Could this explain how dietary restriction works? Hipkiss AR. Ann N Y Acad Sci. 2006 May;1067:361-8.

A strong interaction between serum gamma-glutamyltransferase and obesity on the risk of prevalent type 2 diabetes: results from the Third National Health and Nutrition Examination Survey. Lim JS, Lee DH, Park JY, Jin SH, Jacobs DR Jr. Clin Chem. 2007 Jun;53(6):1092-8. Epub 2007 May 3.

The effects of weight loss and gastric banding on the innate and adaptive immune system in type 2 diabetes and prediabetes. Viardot A, Lord RV, Samaras K. J Clin Endocrinol Metab. 2010 Jun;95(6):2845-50. Epub 2010 Apr 7.

Decrease in peptide methionine sulfoxide reductase in Alzheimer's disease brain. Gabbita SP, Aksenov MY, Lovell MA, Markesbery WR. J Neurochem. 1999 Oct;73(4):1660-6.

Fructose, but not dextrose, accelerates the progression of chronic kidney disease. Gersch MS, Mu W, Cirillo P, Reungjui S, Zhang L, Roncal C, Sautin YY, Johnson RJ, Nakagawa T. Am J Physiol Renal Physiol. 2007 Oct;293(4):F1256-61. Epub 2007 Aug 1.

Hypothesis: could excessive fructose intake and uric acid cause type 2 diabetes? Johnson RJ, Perez-Pozo SE, Sautin YY, Manitius J, Sanchez-Lozada LG, Feig DI, Shafiu M, Segal M, Glassock RJ, Shimada M, Roncal C, Nakagawa T. Endocr Rev. 2009 Feb;30(1):96-116. Epub 2009 Jan 16.

Antibiotics protect against fructose-induced hepatic lipid accumulation in mice: role of endotoxin. Bergheim I, Weber S, Vos M, Krämer S, Volynets V, Kaserouni S, McClain CJ, Bischoff SC. J Hepatol. 2008 Jun;48(6):983-92. Epub 2008 Mar 14.

From inflammation to sickness and depression: when the immune system subjugates the brain. Dantzer R, O'Connor JC, Freund GG, Johnson RW, Kelley KW. Nat Rev Neurosci. 2008 Jan;9(1):46-56.

Regulation of adaptive behaviour during fasting by hypothalamic Foxa2. Silva JP, von Meyenn F, Howell J, Thorens B, Wolfrum C, Stoffel M. Nature. 2009 Dec 3;462(7273):646-50.

Extracellular fatty acid synthase: a possible surrogate biomarker of insulin resistance. Fernandez-Real JM, Menendez JA, Moreno-Navarrete JM, Blüher M, Vazquez-Martin A, Vázquez MJ, Ortega F, Diéguez C, Frühbeck G, Ricart W, Vidal-Puig A. Diabetes. 2010 Jun;59(6):1506-11. Epub 2010 Mar 18.

Extending healthy life span--from yeast to humans. Fontana L, Partridge L, Longo VD. Science. 2010 Apr 16;328(5976):321-6.

Evolutionary origins of obesity. Bellisari A. Obes Rev. 2008 Mar;9(2):165-80.

Epigenetic regulation of Th1 and Th2 cell development. Sanders VM. Brain Behav Immun. 2006 Jul;20(4):317-24. Epub 2005 Oct 11.

Very-low-carbohydrate diets and preservation of muscle mass. Manninen AH. Nutr Metab (Lond). 2006 Jan 31;3:9.

Melanocortin signaling in the CNS directly regulates circulating cholesterol. Perez-Tilve D, Hofmann SM, Basford J, Nogueiras R, Pfluger PT, Patterson JT, Grant E, Wilson-Perez HE, Granholm NA, Arnold M, Trevaskis JL, Butler AA, Davidson WS, Woods SC, Benoit SC, Sleeman MW, DiMarchi RD, Hui DY, Tschöp MH. Nat Neurosci. 2010 Jul;13(7):877-82. Epub 2010 Jun 6.

Clking on PGC-1alpha to inhibit gluconeogenesis. Cantó C, Auwerx J. Cell Metab. 2010 Jan;11(1):6-7.

Cdc2-like kinase 2 is an insulin-regulated suppressor of hepatic gluconeogenesis. Rodgers JT, Haas W, Gygi SP, Puigserver P. Cell Metab. 2010 Jan;11(1):23-34.

Childhood obesity, other cardiovascular risk factors, and premature death. Franks PW, Hanson RL, Knowler WC, Sievers ML, Bennett PH, Looker HC. N Engl J Med. 2010 Feb 11;362(6):485-93.

Cancer as a metabolic disease. Seyfried TN, Shelton LM. Nutr Metab (Lond). 2010 Jan 27;7:7.

Effects of biologics on vascular function and atherosclerosis associated with rheumatoid arthritis. Kerekes G, Soltész P, Dér H, Veres K, Szabó Z, Végvári A, Shoenfeld Y, Szekanecz Z. Ann N Y Acad Sci. 2009 Sep;1173:814-21.

Adjuvant aspirin therapy reduces symptoms of schizophrenia spectrum disorders: results from a randomized, double-blind, placebo-controlled trial. Laan W, Grobbee DE, Selten JP, Heijnen CJ, Kahn RS, Burger H. J Clin Psychiatry. 2010 May;71(5):520-7.

Acylation-stimulating protein/C5L2-neutralizing antibodies alter triglyceride metabolism in vitro and in vivo. Cui W, Paglialunga S, Kalant D, Lu H, Roy C, Laplante M, Deshaies Y, Cianflone K. Am J Physiol Endocrinol Metab. 2007 Dec;293(6):E1482-91. Epub 2007 Aug 21.

Association of adipocyte genes with ASP expression: a microarray analysis of subcutaneous and omental adipose tissue in morbidly obese subjects. MacLaren RE, Cui W, Lu H, Simard S, Cianflone K. BMC Med Genomics. 2010 Jan 27;3:3.

Aldosterone in salt-sensitive hypertension and metabolic syndrome. Fujita T. J Mol Med. 2008 Jun;86(6):729-34. Epub 2008 Apr 25.

Adiponectin and AdipoR1 regulate PGC-1alpha and mitochondria by Ca(2+) and AMPK/SIRT1. Iwabu M, Yamauchi T, Okada-Iwabu M, Sato K, Nakagawa T, Funata M, Yamaguchi M, Namiki S,Nakayama R, Tabata M, Ogata H, Kubota N, Takamoto I, Hayashi YK, Yamauchi N, Waki H,Fukayama M, Nishino I, Tokuyama K, Ueki K, Oike Y, Ishii S, Hirose K, Shimizu T, Touhara K,Kadowaki T. Nature. 2010 Apr 29;464(7293):1313-9. Epub 2010 Mar 31.

ACAT1 gene ablation increases 24(S)-hydroxycholesterol content in the brain and ameliorates amyloid pathology in mice with AD. Bryleva EY, Rogers MA, Chang CC, Buen F, Harris BT, Rousselet E, Seidah NG, Oddo S, LaFerla FM, Spencer TA, Hickey WF, Chang TY. Proc Natl Acad Sci U S A. 2010 Feb 16;107(7):3081-6. Epub 2010 Jan 26.

Cholesterol lowering, sudden cardiac death and mortality. de Lorgeril M, Salen P. Scand Cardiovasc J. 2008 Aug;42(4):264-7.

Women and statin use: a women's health advocacy perspective. Rosenberg H, Allard D. Scand Cardiovasc J. 2008 Aug;42(4):268-73.

The causal role of blood lipids in the aetiology of coronary heart disease--an epidemiologist's perspective. Thelle DS. Scand Cardiovasc J. 2008 Aug;42(4):274-8.

On criticism in bio-medical research--a tribute to Uffe Ravnskov. Folkow B. Scand Cardiovasc J. 2008 Aug;42(4):240-3.

Methionine synthase polymorphism is a risk factor for Alzheimer disease. Beyer K, Lao JI, Latorre P, Riutort N, Matute B, Fernández-Figueras MT, Mate JL, Ariza A. Neuroreport. 2003 Jul 18;14(10):1391-4.

Differential effects of saturated and monounsaturated fats on postprandial lipemia and glucagon-like peptide 1 responses in patients with type 2 diabetes. Thomsen C, Storm H, Holst JJ, Hermansen K. Am J Clin Nutr. 2003 Mar;77(3):605-11.

Grains
Chapter Six: Grains and Leaky Gut

Agrarian diet and diseases of affluence--do evolutionary novel dietary lectins cause leptin resistance? Jönsson T, Olsson S, Ahrén B, Bøg-Hansen TC, Dole A, Lindeberg S. BMC Endocr Disord. 2005 Dec 10;5:10.

Dissociation of the glycaemic and insulinaemic responses to whole and skimmed milk. Hoyt G, Hickey MS, Cordain L. Br J Nutr 2005;93:175-177.

Modulation of immune function by dietary lectins in rheumatoid arthritis. Cordain L, Toohey L, Smith MJ, Hickey MS. Brit J Nutr 2000, 83:207-217.

Cereal grains: humanity's double edged sword. Cordain L. World Rev Nutr Diet 1999; 84:19-73.

Gut flora and bacterial translocation in chronic liver disease. Almeida J, Galhenage S, Yu J, Kurtovic J, Riordan SM. World J Gastroenterol. 2006 Mar 14;12(10):1493-502.

HIV disease progression: immune activation, microbes, and a leaky gut. Douek D. Top HIV Med. 2007 Aug-Sep;15(4):114-7.

HLA genomics in the third millennium. Trowsdale J. Curr Opin Immunol. 2005 Oct;17(5):498-504.

Identification of human zonulin, a physiological modulator of tight junctions, as prehaptoglobin-2. Tripathi A, Lammers KM, Goldblum S, Shea-Donohue T, Netzel-Arnett S, Buzza MS, Antalis TM,Vogel SN, Zhao A, Yang S, Arrietta MC, Meddings JB, Fasano A. Proc Natl Acad Sci U S A. 2009 Sep 29;106(39):16799-804. Epub 2009 Sep 15.

Immune reactivity to a glb1 homologue in a highly wheat-sensitive patient with type 1 diabetes and celiac disease. Mojibian M, Chakir H, MacFarlane AJ, Lefebvre DE, Webb JR, Touchie C, Karsh J, Crookshank JA, Scott FW.Diabetes Care. 2006 May;29(5):1108-10.

Novel immune response to gluten in individuals with schizophrenia. Samaroo D, Dickerson F, Kasarda DD, Green PH, Briani C, Yolken RH, Alaedini A. Schizophr Res. 2010 May;118(1-3):248-55. Epub 2009 Sep 11.

Increased intestinal permeability and tight junction alterations in nonalcoholic fatty liver disease. Miele L, Valenza V, La Torre G, Montalto M, Cammarota G, Ricci R, Mascianà R, Forgione A,Gabrieli ML, Perotti G, Vecchio FM, Rapaccini G, Gasbarrini G, Day CP, Grieco A. Hepatology. 2009 Jun;49(6):1877-87.

Infections and autoimmunity--friends or foes? Kivity S, Agmon-Levin N, Blank M, Shoenfeld Y. Trends Immunol. 2009 Aug;30(8):409-14. Epub 2009 Jul 28.

Autoantibody screen in inflammatory myopathies high prevalence of antibodies to gliadin. Orbach H, Amitai N, Barzilai O, Boaz M, Ram M, Zandman-Goddard G, Shoenfeld Y. Ann N Y Acad Sci. 2009 Sep;1173:174-9.

Innate immunity, epigenetics and autoimmunity in rheumatoid arthritis. Maciejewska Rodrigues H, Jüngel A, Gay RE, Gay S. Mol Immunol. 2009 Nov;47(1):12-8. Epub 2009 Feb 15.

Design and synthesis of potent Quillaja saponin vaccine adjuvants. Adams MM, Damani P, Perl NR, Won A, Hong F, Livingston PO, Ragupathi G, Gin DY. J Am Chem Soc. 2010 Feb 17;132(6):1939-45.

Effect of exclusion diet with nutraceutical therapy in juvenile Crohn's disease. Slonim AE, Grovit M, Bulone L. J Am Coll Nutr. 2009 Jun;28(3):277-85.

Alcohol, intestinal bacterial growth, intestinal permeability to endotoxin, and medical consequences: summary of a symposium. Purohit V, Bode JC, Bode C, Brenner DA, Choudhry MA, Hamilton F, Kang YJ, Keshavarzian A,Rao R, Sartor RB, Swanson C, Turner JR. Alcohol. 2008 Aug;42(5):349-61. Epub 2008 May 27.

Milk--the promoter of chronic Western diseases. Melnik BC. Med Hypotheses. 2009 Jun;72(6):631-9. Epub 2009 Feb 15.

High intakes of milk, but not meat, increase s-insulin and insulin resistance in 8-year-old boys. Hoppe C, Mølgaard C, Vaag A, Barkholt V, Michaelsen KF. Eur J Clin Nutr. 2005 Mar;59(3):393-8.

Multiple sclerosis: could it be an epigenetic disease? Kürtüncü M, Tüzün E. Med Hypotheses. 2008 Dec;71(6):945-7. Epub 2008 Aug 16.

Neurologic presentation of celiac disease. Bushara KO. Gastroenterology. 2005 Apr;128(4 Suppl 1):S92-7.

Intestinal permeability and inflammation in rheumatoid arthritis: effects of non-steroidal anti-inflammatory drugs. Bjarnason I, Williams P, So A, Zanelli GD, Levi AJ, Gumpel JM, Peters TJ, Ansell B. Lancet. 1984 Nov 24;2(8413):1171-4.

Prostaglandins and the induction of food sensitive enteropathy. M McI Gut. 2000 February; 46(2): 154–155.

Reflux oesophagitis in adult coeliac disease: beneficial effect of a gluten free diet. Cuomo A, Romano M, Rocco A, Budillon G, Del Vecchio Blanco C, Nardone G. Gut. 2003 Apr;52(4):514-7.

Shared genetic risk factors for type 1 diabetes and celiac disease. Plenge RM. N Engl J Med. 2008 Dec 25;359(26):2837-8. Epub 2008 Dec 10.

Sporadic cerebellar ataxia associated with gluten sensitivity. Bürk K, Bösch S, Müller CA, Melms A, Zühlke C, Stern M, Besenthal I, Skalej M, Ruck P, Ferber S, Klockgether T, Dichgans J. Brain. 2001 May;124(Pt 5):1013-9.

Surprises from celiac disease. Fasano A. Sci Am. 2009 Aug;301(2):54-61.

Putting the pieces of the puzzle together - a series of hypotheses on the etiology and pathogenesis of type 1 diabetes. Barbeau WE, Bassaganya-Riera J, Hontecillas R. Med Hypotheses. 2007;68(3):607-19. Epub 2006 Oct 11.

The genetics and epigenetics of autoimmune diseases. Hewagama A, Richardson B. J Autoimmun. 2009 Aug;33(1):3-11. Epub 2009 Apr 5.

The genetics of human autoimmune disease. Invernizzi P, Gershwin ME. J Autoimmun. 2009 Nov-Dec;33(3-4):290-9. Epub 2009 Aug 13.

Tissue transglutaminase crosslinks ataxin-1: possible role in SCA1 pathogenesis. D'Souza DR, Wei J, Shao Q, Hebert MD, Subramony SH, Vig PJ. Neurosci Lett. 2006 Nov 27;409(1):5-9. Epub 2006 Oct 11.

A Novel Therapeutic Target in Inflammatory Uveitis: Transglutaminase 2 Inhibitor. Joonhong Sohn, Ju Byung Chae,2 Sun Young Lee, Soo-Youl Kim, and June Gone Kim. Korean J Ophthalmol. 2010 February; 24(1): 29–34.

Intracellular localization and conformational state of transglutaminase 2: implications for cell death. Gundemir S, Johnson GV. PLoS One. 2009 Jul 1;4(7):e6123.

Tissue transglutaminase expression in celiac mucosa: an immunohistochemical study. Gorgun J, Portyanko A, Marakhouski Y, Cherstvoy E. Virchows Arch. 2009 Oct;455(4):363-73. Epub 2009 Sep 12.

Transglutaminases: nature's biological glues. Griffin M, Casadio R, Bergamini CM. Biochem J. 2002 Dec 1;368(Pt 2):377-96.

Serum studies in man after administration of vitamin A acetate and vitamin A alcohol. II. In subjects suffering from disturbances of absorption and digestion. FITZGERALD O, FENNELLY JJ, HINGERTY DJ. Gut. 1962 Mar;3:74-9.

Identification of three wheat globulin genes by screening a Triticum aestivum BAC genomic library with cDNA from a diabetes-associated globulin. Loit E, Melnyk CW, MacFarlane AJ, Scott FW, Altosaar I. BMC Plant Biol. 2009 Jul 17;9:93.

Breath hydrogen and methane responses of men and women to breads made with white flour or whole wheat flours of different particle sizes. Hallfrisch J, Behall KM. J Am Coll Nutr. 1999 Aug;18(4):296-302.

Zonulin upregulation is associated with increased gut permeability in subjects with type 1 diabetes and their relatives. Sapone A, de Magistris L, Pietzak M, Clemente MG, Tripathi A, Cucca F, Lampis R, Kryszak D,Cartenì M, Generoso M, Iafusco D, Prisco F, Laghi F, Riegler G, Carratu R, Counts D, Fasano A. Diabetes. 2006 May;55(5):1443-9.

The gluten connection: the association between schizophrenia and celiac disease. Kalaydjian AE, Eaton W, Cascella N, Fasano A. Acta Psychiatr Scand. 2006 Feb;113(2):82-90.

Dietary gluten and learning to attend to redundant stimuli in rats. Harper DN, Nisbet RH, Siegert RJ. Biol Psychiatry. 1997 Dec 1;42(11):1060-6.

A unifying hypothesis on the development of type 1 diabetes and celiac disease: gluten consumption may be a shared causative factor. Frisk G, Hansson T, Dahlbom I, Tuvemo T. Med Hypotheses. 2008;70(6):1207-9. Epub 2008 Feb 4.

Gluten sensitivity as a neurological illness. Hadjivassiliou M, Grünewald RA, Davies-Jones GA. J Neurol Neurosurg Psychiatry. 2002 May;72(5):560-3.

Headache and CNS white matter abnormalities associated with gluten sensitivity. Hadjivassiliou M, Grünewald RA, Lawden M, Davies-Jones GA, Powell T, Smith CM. Neurology. 2001 Feb 13;56(3):385-8.

Gluten sensitivity in multiple sclerosis: experimental myth or clinical truth? Shor DB, Barzilai O, Ram M, Izhaky D, Porat-Katz BS, Chapman J, Blank M, Anaya JM,Shoenfeld Y. Ann N Y Acad Sci. 2009 Sep;1173:343-9.

Gluten sensitivity in Japanese patients with adult-onset cerebellar ataxia. Ihara M, Makino F, Sawada H, Mezaki T, Mizutani K, Nakase H, Matsui M, Tomimoto H,Shimohama S.Intern Med. 2006;45(3):135-40. Epub 2006 Mar 1.

Gluten ataxia: passive transfer in a mouse model. Boscolo S, Sarich A, Lorenzon A, Passoni M, Rui V, Stebel M, Sblattero D, Marzari R,Hadjivassiliou M, Tongiorgi E. Ann N Y Acad Sci. 2007 Jun;1107:319-28.

Gluten ataxia in perspective: epidemiology, genetic susceptibility and clinical characteristics. Hadjivassiliou M, Grünewald R, Sharrack B, Sanders D, Lobo A, Williamson C, Woodroofe N,Wood N, Davies-Jones A. Brain. 2003 Mar;126(Pt 3):685-91.

Clinical, radiological, neurophysiological, and neuropathological characteristics of gluten ataxia. Hadjivassiliou M, Grünewald RA, Chattopadhyay AK, Davies-Jones GA, Gibson A, Jarratt JA,Kandler RH, Lobo A, Powell T, Smith CM. Lancet. 1998 Nov 14;352(9140):1582-5.

Dietary treatment of gluten ataxia. Hadjivassiliou M, Davies-Jones GA, Sanders DS, Grünewald RA. J Neurol Neurosurg Psychiatry. 2003 Sep;74(9):1221-4.

Autoantibodies in gluten ataxia recognize a novel neuronal transglutaminase. Hadjivassiliou M, Aeschlimann P, Strigun A, Sanders DS, Woodroofe N, Aeschlimann D. Ann Neurol. 2008 Sep;64(3):332-43.

Gliadin IgG antibodies and circulating immune complexes. Eisenmann A, Murr C, Fuchs D, Ledochowski M. Scand J Gastroenterol. 2009;44(2):168-71.

Early impairment of gut function and gut flora supporting a role for alteration of gastrointestinal mucosa in human immunodeficiency virus pathogenesis. Gori A, Tincati C, Rizzardini G, Torti C, Quirino T, Haarman M, Ben Amor K, van Schaik J,Vriesema A, Knol J, Marchetti G, Welling G, Clerici M. J Clin Microbiol. 2008 Feb;46(2):757-8. Epub 2007 Dec 19.

Excitotoxic neuronal death and the pathogenesis of Huntington's disease. Estrada Sánchez AM, Mejía-Toiber J, Massieu L. Arch Med Res. 2008 Apr;39(3):265-76. Pediatrics. 2005 Dec;116(6):e754-9.

Celiac disease: evaluation of the diagnosis and dietary compliance in Canadian children. Rashid M, Cranney A, Zarkadas M, Graham ID, Switzer C, Case S, Molloy M, Warren RE, Burrows V, Butzner JD.

Does rheumatoid arthritis represent an adaptive, thrifty condition? Reser JE, Reser WW. Med Hypotheses. 2010 Jan;74(1):189-94. Epub 2009 Aug 27.

A population-based study of coeliac disease, neurodegenerative and neuroinflammatory diseases. Ludvigsson JF, Olsson T, Ekbom A, Montgomery SM. Aliment Pharmacol Ther. 2007 Jun 1;25(11):1317-27.

Celiac disease. Rubio-Tapia A, Murray JA. Curr Opin Gastroenterol. 2010 Mar;26(2):116-22.

Celiac disease: from gluten to autoimmunity. Briani C, Samaroo D, Alaedini A. Autoimmun Rev. 2008 Sep;7(8):644-50. Epub 2008 Jun 25.

Significance of anti-CCP antibodies in modification of 1987 ACR classification criteria in diagnosis of rheumatoid arthritis. Zhao J, Liu X, Wang Z, Li Z. Clin Rheumatol. 2010 Jan;29(1):33-8. Epub 2009 Oct 15.

Anatomical basis of tolerance and immunity to intestinal antigens. Mowat AM. Nat Rev Immunol. 2003 Apr;3(4):331-41.

Alcohol's role in gastrointestinal tract disorders. Bode C, Bode JC. Alcohol Health Res World. 1997;21(1):76-83.

A type 1 diabetes-related protein from wheat (Triticum aestivum). cDNA clone of a wheat storage globulin, Glb1, linked to islet damage. MacFarlane AJ, Burghardt KM, Kelly J, Simell T, Simell O, Altosaar I, Scott FW. J Biol Chem. 2003 Jan 3;278(1):54-63. Epub 2002 Oct 29.

Gliadin, zonulin and gut permeability: Effects on celiac and non-celiac intestinal mucosa and intestinal cell lines. Drago S, El Asmar R, Di Pierro M, Grazia Clemente M, Tripathi A, Sapone A, Thakar M, Iacono G,Carroccio A, D'Agate C, Not T, Zampini L, Catassi C, Fasano A. Scand J Gastroenterol. 2006 Apr;41(4):408-19.

Supportive Versus Immunosuppressive Therapy of Progressive IgA nephropathy (STOP) IgAN trial: rationale and study protocol. Eitner F, Ackermann D, Hilgers RD, Floege J. J Nephrol. 2008 May-Jun;21(3):284-9.

Fats
Chapter Seven: Fat: Have a Seat, This May Take a Little While

Compared with saturated fatty acids, dietary monounsaturated fatty acids and carbohydrates increase atherosclerosis and VLDL cholesterol levels in LDL receptor-deficient, but not apolipoprotein E-deficient, mice. Merkel M, Velez-Carrasco W, Hudgins LC, Breslow JL. Proc Natl Acad Sci U S A. 2001 Nov 6;98(23):13294-9. Epub 2001 Oct 23.

Saturated fat consumption in ancestral human diets: implications for contemporary intakes. In: Phytochemicals, Nutrient-Gene Interactions. Cordain L., Meskin MS, Bidlack WR, Randolph RK (Eds.), CRC Press (Taylor & Francis Group), 2006, pp. 115-126.

Dietary fat quality and coronary heart disease prevention: a unified theory based on evolutionary, historical, global and modern perspectives. Ramsden CE, Faurot KR, Carrera-Bastos, P, Sperling LS, de Lorgeril M, Cordain L. Curr Treat Options Cardiovasc Med; 2009;11:289-301.

Fatty acid analysis of wild ruminant tissues: Evolutionary implications for reducing diet-related chronic disease. Cordain L, Watkins BA, Florant GL, Kehler M, Rogers L, Li Y. Eur J Clin Nutr, 2002; 56:181-191.

Fat and Fatty Acid Intake and Metabolic Effects in the Human Body. T.A.B. Sanders Ann Nutr Metab 2009;55:162–172.

The Relationship between Dietary Fat and Fatty Acid Intake and Body Weight, Diabetes, and the Metabolic Syndrome. Edward L. Melanson, Arne Astrup, William T. Donahoo. Ann Nutr Metab 2009;55:229–243.

Fish-oil supplement has neutral effects on vascular and metabolic function but improves renal function in patients with Type 2 diabetes mellitus. Wong CY, Yiu KH, Li SW, Lee S, Tam S, Lau CP, Tse HF. Diabet Med. 2010 Jan;27(1):54-60.

Efficacy of Omega-3 Fatty Acids in Children and Adults with IgA Nephropathy Is Dosage- and Size-Dependent. Ronald J. Hogg, Lisa Fitzgibbons, Carolyn Atkins, Nancy Nardelli, and R. Curtis Bay; for the North American IgA Nephropathy Study Group. Clin J Am Soc Nephrol 1: 1167–1172, 2006. doi: 10.2215/CJN.02300606.

Growth and development of preterm infants fed infant formulas containing docosahexaenoic acid and arachidonic acid. Clandinin MT, Van Aerde JE, Merkel KL, Harris CL, Springer MA, Hansen JW, Diersen-Schade DA. J Pediatr. 2005 Apr;146(4):461-8.

Higher de novo synthesized fatty acids and lower o3- and o6-long-chain polyunsaturated fatty acids in umbilical vessels of women with preeclampsia and high fish intakes. Victor J.B. Huiskes a, Remko S. Kuipers a, Francien V. Velzing-Aarts a, D.A. Janneke Dijck-Brouwer a, Jan van der Meulen b, Frits A.J. Muskiet. Prostaglandins, Leukotrienes and Essential Fatty Acids 80 (2009) 101–106

Impaired maternal glucose homeostasis during pregnancy is associated with low status of long-chain polyunsaturated fatty acids. (LCP) and essential fatty acids (EFA) in the fetus. D.A. Janneke Dijck-Brouwera, Mijna Hadders-Algrab, Hylco Bouwstrab, Tama´s Decsic, Gu¨nther Boehmd, Ingrid A. Martinie, E. Rudy Boersmaf, Frits A.J. Muskieta. Prostaglandins, Leukotrienes and Essential Fatty Acids 73 (2005) 85–87.

The insulinotropic potency of fatty acids is influenced profoundly by their chain length and degree of saturation. Stein DT, Stevenson BE, Chester MW, Basit M, Daniels MB, Turley SD, McGarry JD. J Clin Invest. 1997 Jul 15;100(2):398-403.

Intestinally derived lipids: Metabolic regulation and consequences—An overview. Katherine Cianflone, Sabina Paglialunga, Christian Roy. Atherosclerosis Supplements 9 (2008) 63–68.

Determinants of serum triglycerides and high-density lipoprotein choles-terol in traditional Trobriand Islanders: the Kitava Study. Lindeberg S, Ah-rén B, Nilsson A, Cordain L, Nilsson-Ehle P, Vessby B. Scand J Clin Lab Invest. 2003;63(3):175-80.

A randomized trial of a low-carbohydrate diet vs orlistat plus a low-fat diet for weight loss. Yancy WS Jr, Westman EC, McDuffie JR, Grambow SC, Jeffreys AS, Bolton J, Chalecki A,Oddone EZ. Arch Intern Med. 2010 Jan 25;170(2):136-45.

A randomized trial of high-dose compared with low-dose omega-3 fatty acids in severe IgA nephropathy. Donadio JV Jr, Larson TS, Bergstralh EJ, Grande JP. J Am Soc Nephrol. 2001 Apr;12(4):791-9.

Long-chain polyunsaturated fatty acids in maternal and infant nutrition. Muskiet FA, van Goor SA, Kuipers RS, Velzing-Aarts FV, Smit EN, Bouwstra H, Dijck-Brouwer DA, Boersma ER, Hadders-Algra M. Prostaglandins Leukot Es-sent Fatty Acids. 2006 Sep;75(3):135-44. Epub 2006 Jul 28.

Cyclooxygenase-2 generates anti-inflammatory mediators from omega-3 fat-ty acids. Groeger AL, Cipollina C, Cole MP, Woodcock SR, Bonacci G, Rudolph TK, Rudolph V, Freeman BA, Schopfer FJ. Nat Chem Biol. 2010 Jun;6(6):433-41. Epub 2010 May 2.

Long-chain n-3 PUFA: plant v. marine sources. Williams CM, Burdge G. Proc Nutr Soc. 2006 Feb;65(1):42-50.

Polyunsaturated fatty acid status of Dutch vegans and omnivores. Fokkema MR, Brouwer DA, Hasperhoven MB, Hettema Y, Bemelmans WJ, Muskiet FA. Prostaglandins Leukot Essent Fatty Acids. 2000 Nov;63(5):279-85.

Combined treatment with renin-angiotensin system blockers and polyunsatu-rated fatty acids in proteinuric IgA nephropathy: a randomized controlled trial. Ferraro PM, Ferraccioli GF, Gambaro G, Fulignati P, Costanzi S. Nephrol Dial Transplant. 2009 Jan;24(1):156-60. Epub 2008 Aug 6.

Peroxisomal retroconversion of docosahexaenoic acid (22:6(n-3)) to eicosa-pentaenoic acid (20:5(n-3)) studied in isolated rat liver cells. Grønn M, Christensen E, Hagve TA, Christophersen BO. Biochim Biophys Acta. 1991 Jan 4;1081(1):85-91.

Short-term supplementation of low-dose gamma-linolenic acid (GLA), alpha-linolenic acid (ALA), or GLA plus ALA does not augment LCP omega 3 status of Dutch vegans to an appreciable extent. Fokkema MR, Brouwer DA, Hasper-hoven MB, Martini IA, Muskiet FA. Prostaglandins Leukot Essent Fatty Acids. 2000 Nov;63(5):287-92.

Conserved role of SIRT1 orthologs in fasting-dependent inhibition of the lipid/cholesterol regulator SREBP. Walker AK, Yang F, Jiang K, Ji JY, Watts JL, Purushotham A, Boss O, Hirsch ML, Ribich S,Smith JJ, Israelian K, Westphal CH, Rodgers JT, Shioda T, Elson SL, Mulligan P, Najafi-Shoushtari H, Black JC, Thakur JK, Kadyk LC, Whetstine JR, Mostoslavsky R, Puigserver P, Li X, Dyson NJ, Hart AC, Näär AM. Genes Dev. 2010 Jul 1;24(13):1403-17.

The effects on plasma, red cell and platelet fatty acids of taking 12 g/day of ethyl-eicosapentaenoate for 16 months: dihomogammalinolenic, arachidon-ic and docosahexaenoic acids and relevance to Inuit metabolism. Horrobin D, Fokkema MR, Muskiet FA. Prostaglandins Leukot Essent Fatty Acids. 2003 May;68(5):301-4.

Fat and fatty acid terminology, methods of analysis and fat digestion and metabolism: a background review paper. Ratnayake WM, Galli C. Ann Nutr Metab. 2009;55(1-3):8-43. Epub 2009 Sep 15.

Effects of fat and fatty acid intake on inflammatory and immune responses: a critical review. Galli C, Calder PC. Ann Nutr Metab. 2009;55(1-3):123-39. Epub 2009 Sep 15.

Fat intake and CNS functioning: ageing and disease. Crawford MA, Bazinet RP, Sinclair AJ. Ann Nutr Metab. 2009;55(1-3):202-28. Epub 2009 Sep 15.

Background review paper on total fat, fatty acid intake and cancers. Gerber M. Ann Nutr Metab. 2009;55(1-3):140-61. Epub 2009 Sep 15.

Acute or chronic upregulation of mitochondrial fatty acid oxidation has no net effect on whole-body energy expenditure or adiposity. Hoehn KL, Turner N, Swarbrick MM, Wilks D, Preston E, Phua Y, Joshi H, Furler SM, Larance M,Hegarty BD, Leslie SJ, Pickford R, Hoy AJ, Kraegen EW, James DE, Cooney GJ. Cell Metab. 2010 Jan;11(1):70-6.

Dietary fat and coronary heart disease: summary of evidence from prospec-tive cohort and randomised controlled trials. Skeaff CM, Miller J. Ann Nutr Metab. 2009;55(1-3):173-201. Epub 2009 Sep 15.

A diet rich in coconut oil reduces diurnal postprandial variations in circulating tissue plasminogen activator antigen and fasting lipoprotein (a) compared with a diet rich in unsaturated fat in women. Müller H, Lindman AS, Blomfeldt A, Seljeflot I, Pedersen JI. J Nutr. 2003 Nov;133(11):3422-7.

Dietary docosahexaenoic acid as a source of eicosapentaenoic acid in vegetarians and omnivores. Conquer JA, Holub BJ. Lipids. 1997 Mar;32(3):341-5.

Highly purified eicosapentaenoic acid treatment improves nonalcoholic steatohepatitis. Tanaka N, Sano K, Horiuchi A, Tanaka E, Kiyosawa K, Aoyama T. J Clin Gastroenterol. 2008 Apr;42(4):413-8.

Incorporation of n-3 fatty acids into plasma lipid fractions, and erythrocyte membranes and platelets during dietary supplementation with fish, fish oil, and docosahexaenoic acid-rich oil among healthy young men. Vidgren HM, Agren JJ, Schwab U, Rissanen T, Hänninen O, Uusitupa MI. Lipids. 1997 Jul;32(7):697-705.

Differential eicosapentaenoic acid elevations and altered cardiovascular disease risk factor responses after supplementation with docosahexaenoic acid in postmenopausal women receiving and not receiving hormone replacement therapy. Stark KD, Holub BJ. Am J Clin Nutr. 2004 May;79(5):765-73.

Effects of dietary coconut oil on the biochemical and anthropometric profiles of women presenting abdominal obesity. Assunção ML, Ferreira HS, dos Santos AF, Cabral CR Jr, Florêncio TM. Lipids. 2009 Jul;44(7):593-601. Epub 2009 May 13.

Is body size a biomarker for optimizing dosing of omega-3 polyunsaturated fatty acids in the treatment of patients with IgA nephropathy? Donadio JV, Bergstralh EJ, Bibus DM, Grande JP. Clin J Am Soc Nephrol. 2006 Sep;1(5):933-9. Epub 2006 Aug 2.

Endothelium as an organ system. Aird WC. Crit Care Med. 2004 May;32(5 Suppl):S271-9.

Lipid lowering treatment patterns and goal attainment in Nordic patients with hyperlipidemia. Svilaas A, Strandberg T, Eriksson M, Hildebrandt P, Westheim A. Scand Cardiovasc J. 2008 Aug;42(4):279-87.

The fallacies of the lipid hypothesis. Ravnskov U. Scand Cardiovasc J. 2008 Aug;42(4):236-9.

Cholesterol does not cause coronary heart disease in contrast to stress. Rosch PJ. Scand Cardiovasc J. 2008 Aug;42(4):244-9.

End of the road for the diet-heart theory? Werkö L. Scand Cardiovasc J. 2008 Aug;42(4):250-5.

γ-Linolenic acid does not augment long-chain polyunsaturated fatty acid ω-3 status. D. A. J. Brouwe, aY. Hettemaa, J. J. van Doormaalb and F. A. J. Muskieta. Prostaglandins, Leukotrienes and Essential Fatty Acids. Volume 59, Issue 5, November 1998, Pages 329-334.

Sleep
Chapter Eight: Stress and Cortisol or
Why This Book Should Be Titled: Sleep Ya Big Dummy!

Associations between sleep loss and increased risk of obesity and diabetes. Knutson KL, Van Cauter E. Ann N Y Acad Sci. 2008;1129:287-304.

Sleep problems and suicidality in the National Comorbidity Survey Replication. Wojnar M, Ilgen MA, Wojnar J, McCammon RJ, Valenstein M, Brower KJ. J Psychiatr Res. 2009 Feb;43(5):526-31. Epub 2008 Sep 7.

Sleep loss: a novel risk factor for insulin resistance and Type 2 diabetes. Spiegel K, Knutson K, Leproult R, Tasali E, Van Cauter E. J Appl Physiol. 2005 Nov;99(5):2008-19.

Acute partial sleep deprivation increases food intake in healthy men. Brondel L, Romer MA, Nougues PM, Touyarou P, Davenne D. Am J Clin Nutr. 2010 Jun;91(6):1550-9. Epub 2010 Mar 31.

Paradoxical sleep deprivation impairs spatial learning and affects membrane excitability and mitochondrial protein in the hippocampus. Yang RH, Hu SJ, Wang Y, Zhang WB, Luo WJ, Chen JY. Brain Res. 2008 Sep 16;1230:224-32. Epub 2008 Jul 17.

Sleep deprivation and vigilant attention. Lim J, Dinges DF. Ann N Y Acad Sci. 2008;1129:305-22.

Sleep and the epidemic of obesity in children and adults. Van Cauter E, Knutson KL. Eur J Endocrinol. 2008 Dec;159 Suppl 1:S59-66. Epub 2008 Aug 21.

A single night of partial sleep deprivation induces insulin resistance in multiple metabolic pathways in healthy subjects. Donga E, van Dijk M, van Dijk JG, Biermasz NR, Lammers GJ, van Kralingen KW, Corssmit EP,Romijn JA. J Clin Endocrinol Metab. 2010 Jun;95(6):2963-8. Epub 2010 Apr 6.

Roles of circadian rhythmicity and sleep in human glucose regulation. Van Cauter E, Polonsky KS, Scheen AJ. Endocr Rev. 1997 Oct;18(5):716-38.

Risk of breast cancer after night- and shift work: current evidence and ongoing studies in Denmark. Hansen J. Cancer Causes Control. 2006 May;17(4):531-7.

Night shift work, light at night, and risk of breast cancer. Davis S, Mirick DK, Stevens RG. J Natl Cancer Inst. 2001 Oct 17;93(20):1557-62.

Sleep deprivation impairs cAMP signalling in the hippocampus. Vecsey CG, Baillie GS, Jaganath D, Havekes R, Daniels A, Wimmer M, Huang T, Brown KM, Li XY, Descalzi G, Kim SS, Chen T, Shang YZ, Zhuo M, Houslay MD, Abel T. Nature. 2009 Oct 22;461(7267):1122-5.

Long sleep duration and childhood overweight/obesity and body fat. Padez C, Mourao I, Moreira P, Rosado V. Am J Hum Biol. 2009 May-Jun;21(3):371-6.

Epigenetics, evolution, endocrine disruption, health, and disease. Crews D, McLachlan JA. Endocrinology. 2006 Jun;147(6 Suppl):S4-10. Epub 2006 May 11.

Epigenetics and human disease. Jiang YH, Bressler J, Beaudet AL. Annu Rev Genomics Hum Genet. 2004;5:479-510.

Does sleep play a role in memory consolidation? A comparative test. Capellini I, McNamara P, Preston BT, Nunn CL, Barton RA. PLoS One. 2009;4(2):e4609. Epub 2009 Feb 25.

Influence of cortisol status on leptin secretion. Leal-Cerro A, Soto A, Martínez MA, Dieguez C, Casanueva FF. Pituitary. 2001 Jan-Apr;4(1-2):111-6.

Elevated fasting plasma cortisol is associated with ischemic heart disease and its risk factors in people with type 2 diabetes: the Edinburgh type 2 diabetes study. Reynolds RM, Labad J, Strachan MW, Braun A, Fowkes FG, Lee AJ, Frier BM, Seckl JR, Walker BR, Price JF; J Clin Endocrinol Metab. 2010 Apr;95(4):1602-8. Epub 2010 Feb 3.

Circadian timing of food intake contributes to weight gain. Arble DM, Bass J, Laposky AD, Vitaterna MH, Turek FW. Obesity (Silver Spring). 2009 Nov;17(11):2100-2. Epub 2009 Sep 3.

Circadian disruption, shift work and the risk of cancer: a summary of the evidence and studies in Seattle. Davis S, Mirick DK. Cancer Causes Control. 2006 May;17(4):539-45.

Biological clocks and shift work: circadian dysregulation and potential long-term effects. Haus E, Smolensky M. Cancer Causes Control. 2006 May;17(4):489-500.

Association of sleep duration with mortality from cardiovascular disease and other causes for Japanese men and women: the JACC study. Ikehara S, Iso H, Date C, Kikuchi S, Watanabe Y, Wada Y, Inaba Y, Tamakoshi A Sleep. 2009 Mar 1;32(3):295-301.

Exercise
Chapter Nine: Ancestral Fitness

Exercise in the fasted state facilitates fibre type-specific intramyocellular lipid breakdown and stimulates glycogen resynthesis in humans. K De Bock,1 EA Richter,2 AP Russell,3 BO Eijnde,1 W Derave,1 M Ramaekers,1 E Koninckx,1 B Léger,3 J Verhaeghe,4 and P Hespel1. J Physiol. 2005 April 15; 564(Pt 2): 649–660. Published online 2005 February 10. doi: 10.1113/jphysiol.2005.083170.

Evolutionary aspects of exercise. Cordain L, Gotshall RW, Eaton SB. Department of Exercise and Sport Science, Colorado State University, Fort Collins, USA. World Rev Nutr Diet. 1997;81:49-60.

Physical activity, energy expenditure and fitness: an evolutionary perspective. Cordain, L., Gotshall, R.W. and Eaton, S.B. International Journal of Sports Medicine 1998; 19:328-335.

Exercise type and intensity in relation to coronary heart disease in men. Tanasescu M, Leitzmann MF, Rimm EB, Willett WC, Stampfer MJ, Hu FB. JAMA. 2002 Oct 23-30;288(16):1994-2000.

Lack of adequate appreciation of physical exercise's complexities can pre-empt appropriate design and interpretation in scientific discovery. Booth FW, Laye MJ. J Physiol. 2009 Dec 1;587(Pt 23):5527-39. Epub 2009 Sep 1.

Reduced physical activity and risk of chronic disease: the biology behind the consequences. Booth FW, Laye MJ, Lees SJ, Rector RS, Thyfault JP. Eur J Appl Physiol. 2008 Mar;102(4):381-90. Epub 2007 Nov 7.

Exercise and gene expression: physiological regulation of the human genome through physical activity. Booth FW, Chakravarthy MV, Spangenburg EE. J Physiol. 2002 Sep 1;543(Pt 2):399-411.

Waging war on modern chronic diseases: primary prevention through exercise biology. Booth FW, Gordon SE, Carlson CJ, Hamilton MT. J Appl Physiol. 2000 Feb;88(2):774-87.

Intramuscular triacylglycerol, glycogen and acetyl group metabolism during 4 h of moderate exercise in man. Watt MJ, Heigenhauser GJ, Dyck DJ, Spriet LL. J Physiol. 2002 Jun 15;541(Pt 3):969-78.

Six sessions of sprint interval training increases muscle oxidative potential and cycle endurance capacity in humans. Burgomaster KA, Hughes SC, Heigenhauser GJ, Bradwell SN, Gibala MJ. J Appl Physiol. 2005 Jun;98(6):1985-90. Epub 2005 Feb 10.

Evolutionary aspects of exercise. Cordain, L., Gotshall, R.W., Eaton, S.B. World Rev Nutr Diet 1997; 81:49-60.

Energy deficit after exercise augments lipid mobilization but does not contribute to the exercise-induced increase in insulin sensitivity. Newsom SA, Schenk S, Thomas KM, Harber MP, Knuth ND, Goldenberg N, Horowitz JF. J Appl Physiol. 2010 Mar;108(3):554-60. Epub 2009 Dec 31.

Timing protein intake increases energy expenditure 24 h after resistance training. Hackney KJ, Bruenger AJ, Lemmer JT. Med Sci Sports Exerc. 2010 May;42(5):998-1003.

Fundamental questions about genes, inactivity, and chronic diseases. Booth FW, Lees SJ. Physiol Genomics. 2007 Jan 17;28(2):146-57. Epub 2006 Oct 10.

Influence of dietary carbohydrate intake on the free testosterone: cortisol ratio responses to short-term intensive exercise training. Lane AR, Duke JW, Hackney AC. Eur J Appl Physiol. 2010 Apr;108(6):1125-31. Epub 2009 Dec 20.

Control of gene expression in adult skeletal muscle by changes in the inherent level of contractile activity. Booth FW, Kirby CR. Biochem Soc Trans. 1991 Apr;19(2):374-8.

Metabolic signatures of exercise in human plasma. Lewis GD, Farrell L, Wood MJ, Martinovic M, Arany Z, Rowe GC, Souza A, Cheng S, McCabe EL,Yang E, Shi X, Deo R, Roth FP, Asnani A, Rhee EP, Systrom DM, Semigran MJ, Vasan RS, Carr SA, Wang TJ, Sabatine MS, Clish CB, Gerszten RE. Sci Transl Med. 2010 May 26;2(33):33ra37.

A moderate serving of high-quality protein maximally stimulates skeletal muscle protein synthesis in young and elderly subjects. Symons TB, Sheffield-Moore M, Wolfe RR, Paddon-Jones D. J Am Diet Assoc. 2009 Sep;109(9):1582-6.

Transcriptional regulation of gene expression in human skeletal muscle during recovery from exercise. HENRIETTE PILEGAARD, GEORGE A. ORDWAY, BENGT SALTIN, AND P. DARRELL NEUFER3. Am J Physiol Endocrinol Metab 279: E806 – E814, 2000.

Promoting training adaptations through nutritional interventions. JOHN A. HAWLEY1, KEVIN D. TIPTON2, & MINDY L. MILLARD-STAFFORD3. Journal of Sports Sciences, July 2006; 24(7): 709 – 721.

Resistance Training Reduces Fasted- and Fed-State Leucine Turnover and Increases Dietary Nitrogen Retention in Previously. Untrained Young Men. Daniel R. Moore,2,3 Nicole C. Del Bel,2,3 Kevin I. Nizi,2,3 Joseph W. Hartman,3 Jason E. Tang,3 David Armstrong,4 and Stuart M. Phillips3* The Journal of Nutrition.

Effects of moderate-intensity endurance and high-intensity intermittent training on anaerobic capacity and VO2max. Tabata I, Nishimura K, Kouzaki M, Hirai Y, Ogita F, Miyachi M, Yamamoto K. Med Sci Sports Exerc. 1996 Oct;28(10):1327-30.

Implementation
Chapter Ten: Implementing the Paleo Solution: It's Easy, Really

Realigning our 21st century diet and lifestyle with our hunter-gatherer genetic identity. Abuissa H, O'Keefe JH, Cordain, L. Directions Psych 2005;25: SR1-SR10.

Origins and evolution of the western diet: Health implications for the 21st century. Loren Cordain, S. Boyd Eaton, Anthony Sebastian, Neil Mann, Staffan Lindeberg, Bruce A. Watkins, James H. O'Keefe, Janette Brand Miller. Am J Clin Nutr 2005;81:341-54.

Cardiovascular disease resulting from a diet and lifestyle at odds with our Paleolithic genome: how to become a 21st-century hunter-gatherer. O'Keefe JH Jr, Cordain L. Mayo Clin Proc 2004 Jan;79(1):101-8.

Biological and clinical potential of a Paleolithic diet. Lindeberg S, Cordain L, and Eaton SB. J Nutri Environ Med 2003; 13(3):149-160.

The paradoxical nature of hunter-gatherer diets: Meat based, yet non-atherogenic. Cordain L, Eaton SB, Brand Miller J, Mann N, Hill K. Eur J Clin Nutr 2002; 56 (suppl 1):S42-S52.

The nutritional characteristics of a contemporary diet based upon Paleolithic food groups. Cordain L. J Am Nutraceut Assoc 2002; 5:15-24.

Fatty acid composition and energy density of foods available to African hominids: evolutionary implications for human brain development. Cordain L, Watkins BA, Mann NJ. World Rev Nutr Diet 2001, 90:144-161.

An evolutionary foundation for health promotion. Eaton SB, Cordain L, Eaton SB. World Rev Nutr Diet 2001; 90:5-12.

Plant to animal subsistence ratios and macronutrient energy estimations in world wide hunter-gatherer diets. Cordain L, Brand Miller J, Eaton SB, Mann N, Holt SHA, Speth JD. Am J Clin Nutr 2000, 71:682-92.

Increased meal frequency does not promote greater weight loss in subjects who were prescribed an 8-week equi-energetic energy-restricted diet. Cameron JD, Cyr MJ, Doucet E. Br J Nutr. 2010 Apr;103(8):1098-101. Epub 2009 Nov 30.

A review of fatty acid profiles and antioxidant content in grass-fed and grain-fed beef. Daley CA, Abbott A, Doyle PS, Nader GA, Larson S. Nutr J. 2010 Mar 10;9:10.

Carbohydrate restriction as the default treatment for type 2 diabetes and metabolic syndrome. Feinman RD, Volek JS. Scand Cardiovasc J. 2008 Aug;42(4):256-63.

Chapter Eleven: Tracking Your Progress

Coronary artery disease prognosis and C-reactive protein levels improve in proportion to percent lowering of low-density lipoprotein. O'Keefe JH Jr, Cordain L, Jones PG, Abuissa H. Am J Cardiol. 2006 Jul 1;98(1):135-9. Epub 2006 May 9.

Optimal low-density lipoprotein is 50 to 70 mg/dl: lower is better and physiologically normal. O'Keefe JH Jr, Cordain L, Harris WH, Moe RM, Vogel R. J Am Coll Cardiol. 2004 Jun 2;43(11):2142-6.

Effects of a short-term intervention with a paleolithic diet in healthy volunteers. Osterdahl M, Kocturk T, Koochek A, Wändell PE. Eur J Clin Nutr. 2008 May;62(5):682-5. Epub 2007 May 16.

Obesity, waist-hip ratio and hunter-gatherers. Wood LE. BJOG. 2006 Oct;113(10):1110-6.

Said another way: stroke, evolution, and the rainforests: an ancient approach to modern health care. Collins C. Nurs Forum. 2007 Jan-Mar;42(1):39-44.

Hypertension, the Kuna, and the epidemiology of flavanols. McCullough ML, Chevaux K, Jackson L, Preston M, Martinez G, Schmitz HH, Coletti C, Campos H, Hollenberg NK. J Cardiovasc Pharmacol. 2006;47 Suppl 2:S103-9; discussion 119-21.

Cardiovascular disease resulting from a diet and lifestyle at odds with our Paleolithic genome: how to become a 21st-century hunter-gatherer. O'Keefe JH Jr, Cordain L. Mayo Clin Proc. 2004 Jan;79(1):101-8.

Optimal low-density lipoprotein is 50 to 70 mg/dl. Lower is better and physiologically normal. O'Keefe JH, Cordain L, Harris, WH, Moe RM, Vogel R. J Am Coll Cardiol 2004;43: 2142-6.

Determinants of serum triglycerides and high-density lipoprotein cholesterol in traditional Trobriand Islanders: the Kitava Study. Lindeberg S, Ahren B, Nilsson A, Cordain L, Nilsson-Ehle P, Vessby B. Scand J Clin Lab Invest 2003; 63: 175-180.

Glycated hemoglobin, diabetes, and cardiovascular risk in nondiabetic adults. Selvin E, Steffes MW, Zhu H, Matsushita K, Wagenknecht L, Pankow J, Coresh J, Brancati FL. N Engl J Med. 2010 Mar 4;362(9):800-11.

Cholesteryl Ester Transfer Protein Polymorphism (TaqIB) Associates With Risk in Postinfarction Patients With High C-Reactive Protein and High-Density Lipoprotein Cholesterol Levels. Corsetti JP, Ryan D, Rainwater DL, Moss AJ, Zareba W, Sparks CE. Arterioscler Thromb Vasc Biol. 2010 Aug;30(8):1657-64. Epub 2010 May 20.

Chapter Twelve: Thirty-Day Meal Plan

The New Vitamin D
What's Putting Fresh Emphasis on Lab Measurements? By Gina Rollins. December 2007 Clinical Laboratory News: The New Vitamin D. December 2007: Volume 33, Number 12.

Can Vitamin D Reduce Total Mortality? Edward Giovannucci, MD, ScD. Arch Intern Med. 2007;167(16):1709-1710.

Vitamin D supplementation. Bruce Eveleigh, MD. Can Fam Physician. Vol. 53, No. 9, September 2007, p.1435. Copyright © 2007 by The College of Family Physicians of Canada.

THE CLINICAL IMPORTANCE OF VITAMIN D (CHOLECALCIFEROL): A PARADIGM SHIFT WITH IMPLICATIONS FOR ALL HEALTHCARE PROVIDERS. Alex Vasquez, Gilbert Manso, , John Cannell, Alternative Therapies, Sept/Oct 2004. VOL. 10.NO. 5.

Scaling of the Mammalian Brain: the Maternal Energy Hypothesis. RD Martin. News Physiol Sci 11: 149-156, 1996;1548-9213/96.

Vitamin D status and its relation to muscle mass and muscle fat in young women. Gilsanz V, Kremer A, Mo AO, Wren TA, Kremer R. J Clin Endocrinol Metab. 2010 Apr;95(4):1595-601. Epub 2010 Feb 17.

Vitamin D decreases respiratory syncytial virus induction of NF-kappaB-linked chemokines and cytokines in airway epithelium while maintaining the antiviral state. Hansdottir S, Monick MM, Lovan N, Powers L, Gerke A, Hunninghake GW. J Immunol. 2010 Jan 15;184(2):965-74. Epub 2009 Dec 11.

Regulation of bile acid synthesis by fat-soluble vitamins A and D. Schmidt DR, Holmstrom SR, Fon Tacer K, Bookout AL, Kliewer SA, Mangelsdorf DJ. Department of Pharmacology and Howard Hughes Medical Institute, University of Texas. J Biol Chem. 2010 May 7;285(19):14486-94. Epub 2010 Mar 16.

Levels of vitamin D and cardiometabolic disorders: systematic review and meta-analysis. Parker J, Hashmi O, Dutton D, Mavrodaris A, Stranges S, Kandala NB, Clarke A, Franco OH. Maturitas. 2010 Mar;65(3):225-36. Epub 2009 Dec 23.

Autism and vitamin D. Cannell JJ. Med Hypotheses. 2008;70(4):750-9. Epub 2007 Oct 24.

Supplementation with an algae source of docosahexaenoic acid increases (n-3) fatty acid status and alters selected risk factors for heart disease in vegetarian subjects. Conquer JA, Holub BJ. J Nutr. 1996 Dec;126(12):3032-9.

Reactive oxygen species enhance insulin sensitivity. Loh K, Deng H, Fukushima A, Cai X, Boivin B, Galic S, Bruce C, Shields BJ, Skiba B, Ooms LM,Stepto N, Wu B, Mitchell CA, Tonks NK, Watt MJ, Febbraio MA, Crack PJ, Andrikopoulos S,Tiganis T. Cell Metab. 2009 Oct;10(4):260-72.

Probiotics improve high fat diet-induced hepatic steatosis and insulin resistance by increasing hepatic NKT cells. Ma X, Hua J, Li Z. J Hepatol. 2008 Nov;49(5):821-30. Epub 2008 Jun 30.

Multivitamin use and risk of cancer and cardiovascular disease in the Women's Health Initiative cohorts. Neuhouser ML, Wassertheil-Smoller S, Thomson C, Aragaki A, Anderson GL, Manson JE,Patterson RE, Rohan TE, van Horn L, Shikany JM, Thomas A, LaCroix A, Prentice RL. Arch Intern Med. 2009 Feb 9;169(3):294-304.

Oral magnesium supplementation improves insulin sensitivity and metabolic control in type 2 diabetic subjects: a randomized double-blind controlled trial. Rodríguez-Morán M, Guerrero-Romero F. Diabetes Care. 2003 Apr;26(4):1147-52.

Magnesium deficiency produces insulin resistance and increased thromboxane synthesis. Nadler JL, Buchanan T, Natarajan R, Antonipillai I, Bergman R, Rude R. Hypertension. 1993 Jun;21(6 Pt 2):1024-9.

How to optimize vitamin D supplementation to prevent cancer, based on cellular adaptation and hydroxylase enzymology. Vieth R. Anticancer Res. 2009 Sep;29(9):3675-84.

High fructose consumption combined with low dietary magnesium intake may increase the incidence of the metabolic syndrome by inducing inflammation. Rayssiguier Y, Gueux E, Nowacki W, Rock E, Mazur A. Magnes Res. 2006 Dec;19(4):237-43.

Erythrocyte fatty acid profiles can predict acute non-fatal myocardial infarction. Park Y, Lim J, Lee J, Kim SG. Br J Nutr. 2009 Nov;102(9):1355-61. Epub 2009 Jun 9.

Why are immigrants at increased risk for psychosis? Vitamin D insufficiency, epigenetic mechanisms, or both? Dealberto MJ. Med Hypotheses. 2007;68(2):259-67. Epub 2006 Oct 2.

Betaine in human nutrition. Craig SA. Am J Clin Nutr. 2004 Sep;80(3):539-49.

Antioxidants prevent health-promoting effects of physical exercise in humans. Ristow M, Zarse K, Oberbach A, Klöting N, Birringer M, Kiehntopf M, Stumvoll M, Kahn CR, Blüher M. Proc Natl Acad Sci U S A. 2009 May 26;106(21):8665-70. Epub 2009 May 11.

Antioxidant supplements for prevention of mortality in healthy participants and patients with various diseases. Bjelakovic G, Nikolova D, Gluud LL, Simonetti RG, Gluud C. Cochrane Database Syst Rev. 2008 Apr 16;(2):CD007176.

Association of A1C levels with vitamin D status in U.S. adults: data from the National Health and Nutrition Examination Survey. Kositsawat J, Freeman VL, Gerber BS, Geraci S. Diabetes Care. 2010 Jun;33(6):1236-8. Epub 2010 Mar 9.